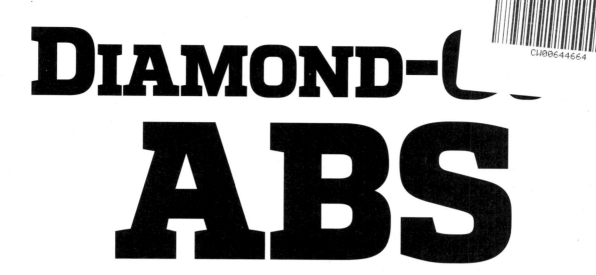

DIAMOND-CUT ABS

HOW TO ENGINEER THE ULTIMATE SIX-PACK— MINIMALIST METHODS FOR MAXIMAL RESULTS

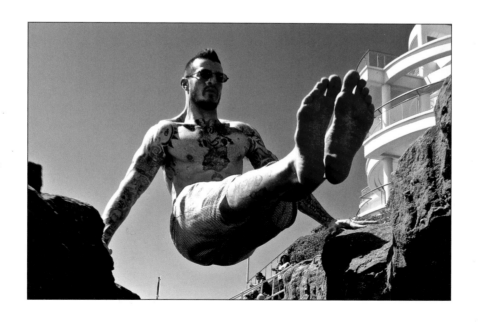

By Danny Kavadlo

DIAMOND-CUT ABS

By Danny Kavadlo

ISBN 10: 0-938045-64-4   ISBN 13: 978-0-938045-64-9

This edition first published in October, 2014
Printed in China

BOOK DESIGN AND COVER: Derek Brigham, site: www.dbrigham.com

PHOTOGRAPHY: Al Kavadlo, Jennifer Regan-Kavadlo, Wilson Cash Kavadlo, Adrienne Harvey, Matt Mendelsohn, Jordan Perlson, Chia Messina, Angelo Grinceri, Rosalia Chann, Naturally Intense Photography, Robert Rimoczi, Grace Menendez, Tamar Kaye, Matthew Palfrey, Simon Abrams, Stephanie Roth-Mizrahi, Abdiel Munoz, Magnus Unnar & Kadri Kurgunm.

MODELS: Beth Andrews, Jasmine Brooks, Rosalia Chann, Alfred DiGrazia, Angelo Gala, the General from U Tough Bootcamp, Ashley Hafstead, Angelo Grinceri, Adrian Harrington, Adrienne Harvey, Al Kavadlo, Errick McAdams, Grace Menendez, Metz, Jennifer Noland, Allegra Poggio, Jennifer Regan-Kavadlo, Rick Richards, Kevin Richardson, Patrick "Packy" Sweeney, Parichart Thepvongs, Tonny Uy, Adam Von Rothfelder, Sylwia Wiesenberg & Chunhua Yang.

FEATURED TATTOOS: Back and chest pieces by Louis Andrew, Buddha belly by Benny, Water by Coney Island Vinnie.

Flying Kavadlo Bros. "Alive" Banner by Marie Roberts (www.ConeyIsland.com)

"Danny The Genie" & "Exercise Your Demons" Illustrations by Mark Robinson (www.eatsharks.com.au)

DISCLAIMER: The author and publisher of this material are not responsible in any manner whatsoever for any injury that may occur through following the instructions contained in this material. The activities, physical and otherwise, described herein for informational purposes only, may be too strenuous or dangerous for some people and the reader(s) should consult a physician before engaging in them.

"The shortest answer is doing the thing."

–Ernest Hemingway

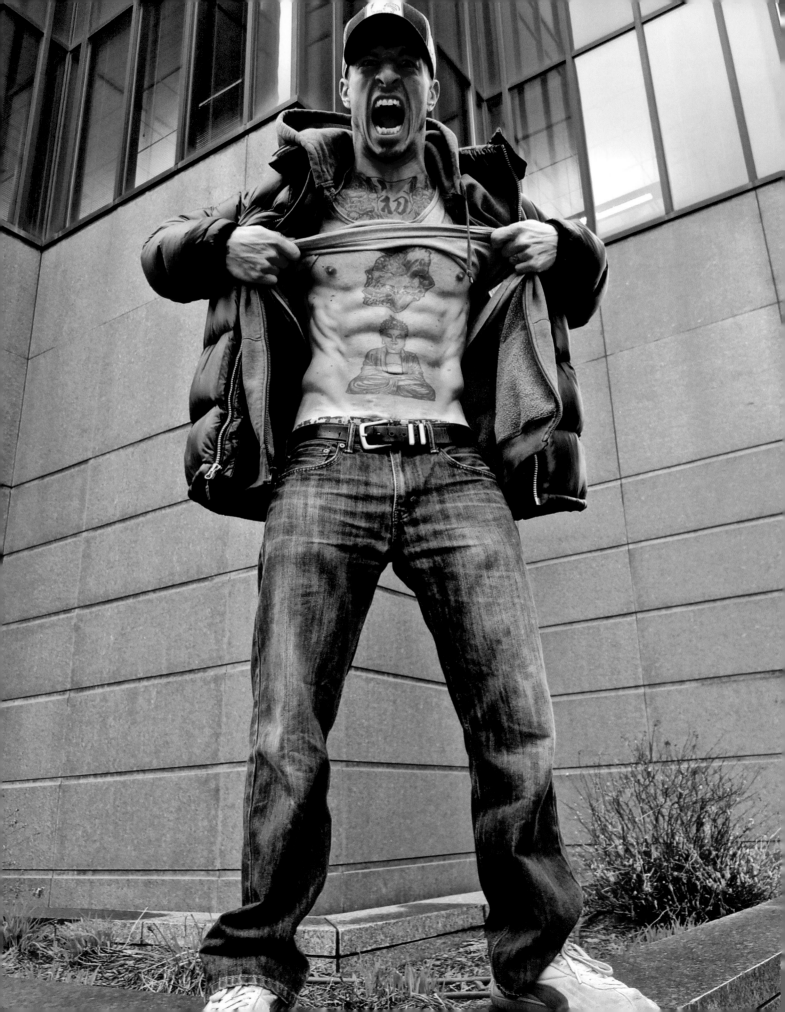

TABLE OF CONTENTS

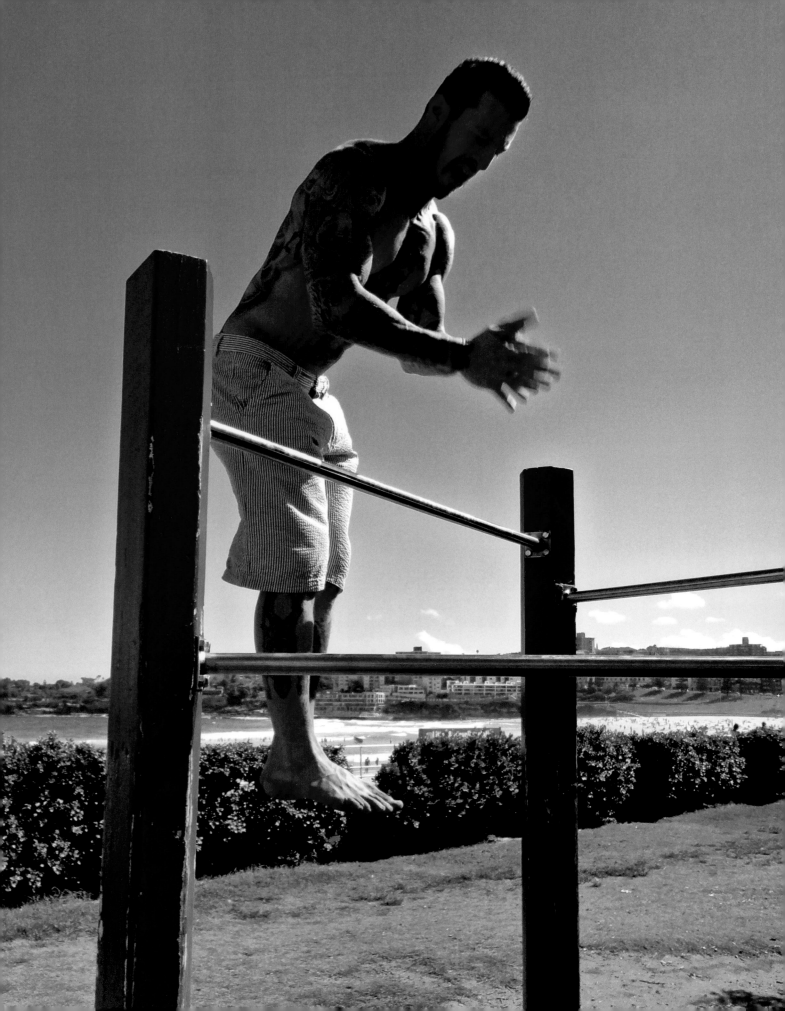

FOREWORD

By Paul "Coach" Wade
Author of *Convict Conditioning*

Anyone who has ever read a Batman comic knows how the young Bruce Wayne travelled the world looking for the greatest masters...those men and women who could teach him how to become the very best, in the quickest time possible, in the arts and disciplines he needed to learn.

Let me say this—if Bruce Wayne had needed to learn how to train his midsection—to get it as lean, strong, athletic and goddam stacked as he humanly could—he would have headed from Gotham straight to New York City and worked with Danny Kavadlo.

Danny is one of the greatest calisthenics coaches on the planet. (And by that, I don't mean top *100*. More like top *3*.) I know how Danny thinks; I've seen how Danny works; I've seen the statistics; I've seen the results. The athletes who have trained under Danny have made such progress in such short time that to an outside eye—to someone who doesn't really understand

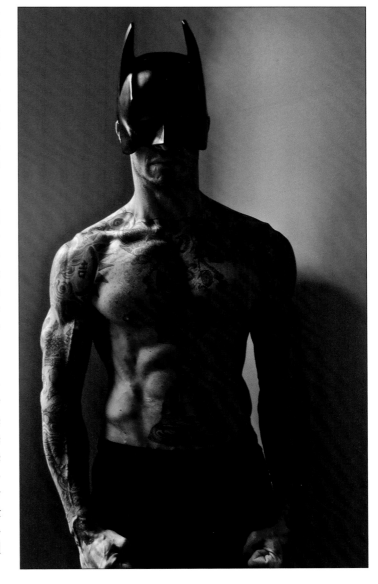

what's going on—it almost seems like *magic*. And this is when he works with athletes who are already considered advanced by normal standards.

Normally, to get the kind of results Danny delivers, you'd have to go to New York to train under his guidance (if you could get a slot!) or attend one of the international *Progressive Calisthenics Certifications* (PCC) where Danny instructs as a Master PCC. (At the time of writing, Danny is one of only two men ever to be granted *Master* PCC teaching status by Dragon Door. The other is Danny's brother, the world-famous Al Kavadlo.)

Luckily for the rest of us, Danny has agreed to put his knowledge on midsection training into a manual—this manual: ***Diamond-Cut Abs***.

You might be thinking: *But Coach, there are plenty of ab-training books on the shelves. Scores. Hundreds, maybe. So what's so special about this one?* Happy you asked, pilgrim.

There is an image in this book which really rings true for me. The image is of Danny—dressed as Morpheus, from the Matrix—offering the reader a blue fruit, or a red fruit. In the movie, Morpheus offers Neo a more drastic choice: the choice to go back to sleep and live as a slave in a fantasy world, or the knowledge of reality and hidden truths, which will be sometimes difficult, but ultimately far more productive and rewarding. This is a perfect metaphor for current abdominal training.

Most people outside the fitness industry don't realize it, but modern abdominal training methods—the kind you find in 99.9% of books and articles—are smoke and mirrors. They're a fantasy, like the Matrix. Folks are told they need this or that supplement (which doesn't work); they are told a load of complete shit about diet and nutrition (stuff which may work for steroid users, but not normal people); and, worst of all, the drills people are given as training exercises are typically worse than useless. Most modern abdominal exercises evolved (or *devolved*) in the sixties, when steroids like Dianabol and Primobalan hit the scene. These drugs made *all* the tissues of the body highly responsive to growth stimulation—even the abs. Juicing bodybuilders got worried that traditional hard, productive abdominal training methods would cause the waist to grow, thus ruining the V-taper so desired in competition. They began to discard the older, functional, strength-producing, truly athletic exercises, choosing to develop methods which could help them tense their abs on stage, *but which would be ineffective at actually building muscle and compound strength*. Ab work became built around light, high-repetition isolation exercises, based on tensing and toning the six-pack.

In other words, most modern bodybuilding methods are *designed* to be inefficient! But at least they're easy to do, right..? Hell, these days you might not even need to actually do anything…you can buy belts now that freeze or zap the fat off your gut while you're on the can. Or, if you prefer, you can buy a million-and-one fat-burning supplements online, right?

Yep. And if you think that stuff will actually give you a six-pack you might want to check the dictionary—they left out the word *gullible*!

If you are smart enough to want nothing to do with this charade, then *Diamond-Cut Abs* is the red pill. In these pages you will learn the painful reality about perfecting the midsection. It may be more difficult than the silly stuff in other books, it may be more old-school than the made-up crap you see on infomercials, but it's also a truckload more rewarding—because it works, big time. I can promise you that.

Danny is not a bodybuilder in the traditional sense. He learned his craft from bodyweight training, where abs cannot be an afterthought—hell, even push-ups and pull-ups are impossible if your abs aren't in shape. (A recent scientific study showed that abs are worked harder during pull-ups than during any other exercise!) This manual condenses decades of agonizing lessons and insight into the *best book on ab-training ever written*. Hands down.

I can promise you that, although it might be challenging, the journey will also be fun. Despite Danny's encyclopedic knowledge, he doesn't take himself too seriously, and he's blessed with a sense of humor.

So whaddya say kid? Do you want the strongest, healthiest, most awesome abdominals of your life? Then grab the red pill.

Let's see how deep this rabbit-hole goes.

Paul Wade 2014

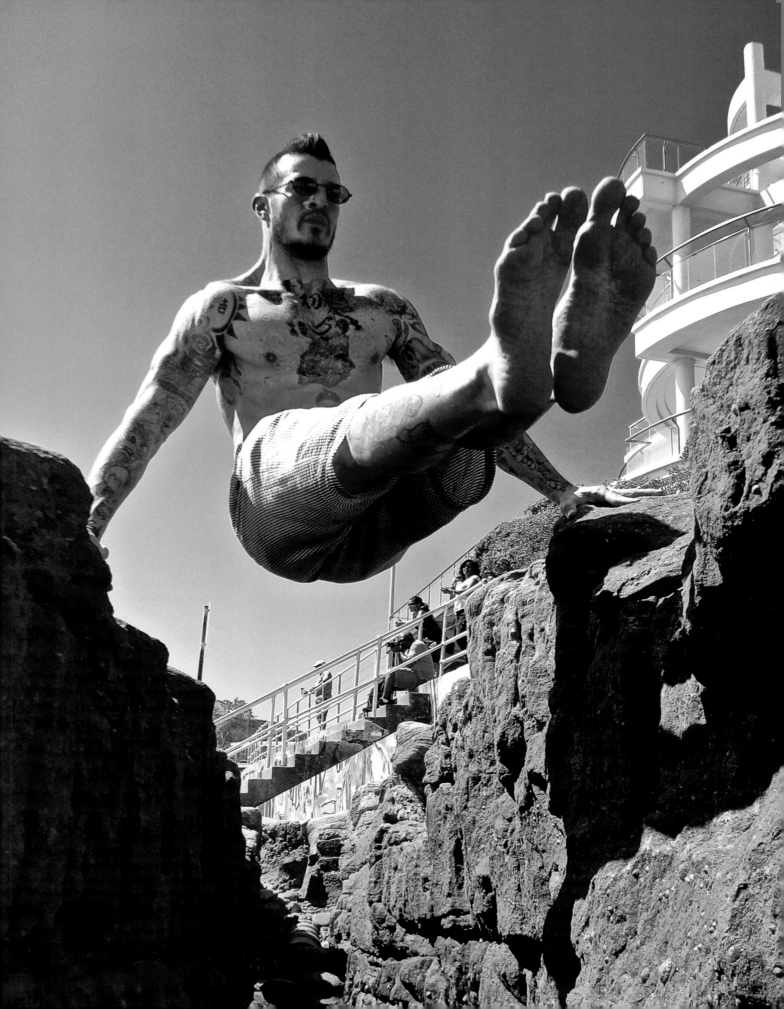

PART I

AN ABS ODYSSEY

"Once you make a decision, the universe conspires to make it happen."

–Ralph Waldo Emerson

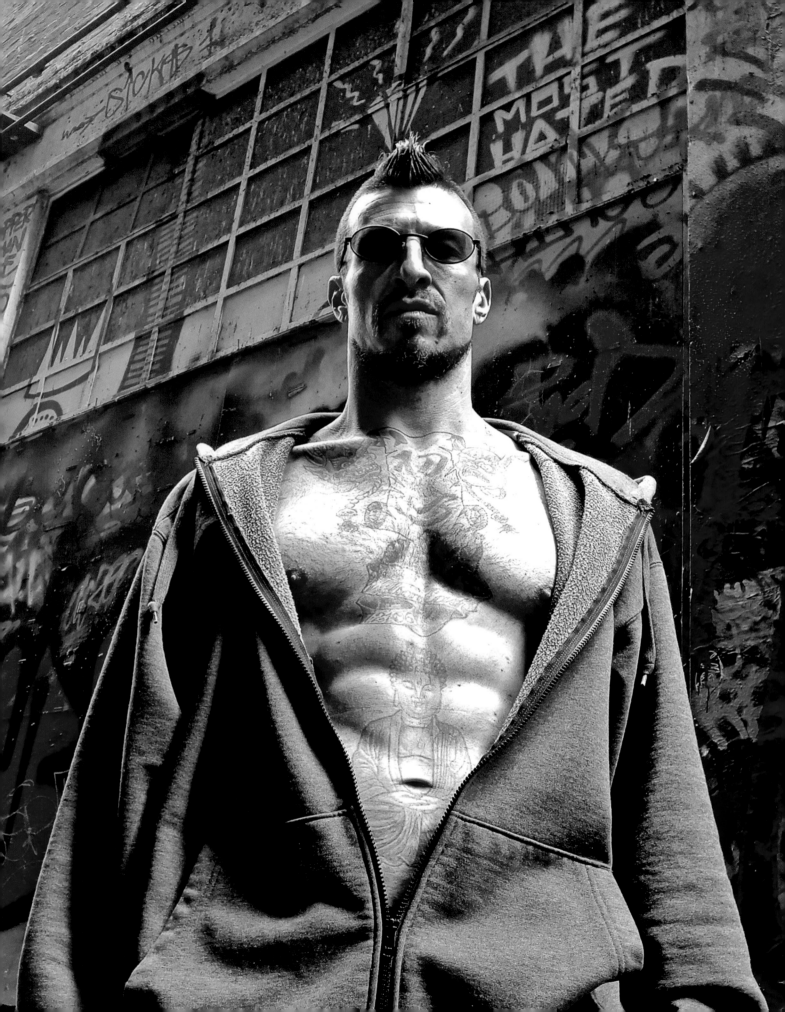

CHAPTER 1

CULTURAL OBSESSION

The universe is enormous. Impossibly large. I could not begin to tell you what is out there. I barely know what's happening here. But I can state the following with supreme certainty and utmost confidence: We, the "civilized" people of planet Earth, have an obsession with abs. That's a fact.

Almost everywhere you look in popular culture, you will find attractive, enticing images of abs. If I turn on the TV and see a bare midsection, chances are it's a fit midsection. Slim, trim, lean and sculpted. How nice.

It's the same thing with the magazine covers, advertisements and billboards. Look at our idols, our heroes, our athletes and movie stars. Just about all of them have one thing in common: abs.

Naturally, this indisputable anthropological fact is even more exaggerated in the world of fitness and fitness-related products. In general, there are an awful lot of workout programs, equipment, apps and DVD's flooding the marketplace. It seems that a disproportionately large number of these products and methods focus on the abdominal area. Considering the effort, function, and yields of training to achieve firm, toned, sexy abs, as compared to the yields of, say, training legs, it would seem logical that there would be more products about squatting than there are about abs, wouldn't it? But we don't have to look any farther than the internet or late-night infomercials to see this is *ab-solutely* not the case.

This principle remains true when I walk into the bookstore. (Yes, I still walk into brick and mortar bookstores.) There are diet manuals, cook books, "new" eating styles, running manifestos, weight training instructions, calisthenic workouts and literature about arms and butt. But like the TV, there seems to be more abs-related material than any other body part. Each has a "proven" method that claims to work for everyone in all situations.

So why this book? Why now? Did I want to be part of an already over-crowded marketplace?

No, not necessarily.

But this book *had* to be written. What I'd been seeing appeared to miss a very important *point* and a seemingly obvious *truth*.

The Point is: Everybody is different (and every *body* is different--think about it). We live in a day and age where fake images of "perfection" are crammed into our eye sockets from youth, and we're instilled with the perverse pursuit of this fantasy, using theoretical formulas to morph into said images. Ours is a crazy world of half-fiction--it's hard to identify what is real and what is not. Magazine covers chop heads off their models and super-impose them onto stretched out bodies. Movie star images and album covers perpetuate fakery and visual manipulation that far surpass my preferred methods of good lighting and no breakfast. It's borderline animation. Fantasyland. In the industry, it's called "idealized". We can never move forward until we accept ourselves and accept what is real. I mean it.

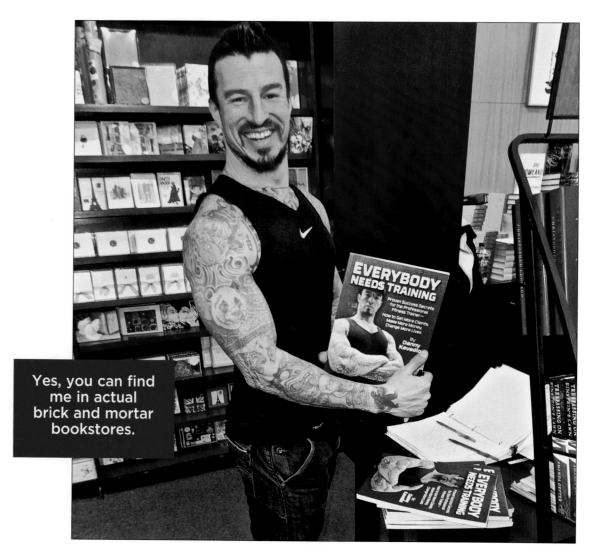

Yes, you can find me in actual brick and mortar bookstores.

The Truth is: Not every program works the same for everybody. This assertion holds up with exercise as well as eating style. Yes, there are accurate generalizations and overall adjustments that hold true for all types, like eat less junk and workout more, but there is no "program" that works identically for everyone. The sooner we make that clear the better. (We will revisit this subject repeatedly.) Your abs are your own. No matter what exercises I do, how hard I train or what I eat, my abs will never look exactly like Brad Pitt's, much the same way my lips will never look exactly like Angelina Jolie's. They can still look amazing, but they'll always look like me. It's still important to remember, however, that just because genetics play a role in the shape of your musculature, any healthy individual can still achieve their own set of off-the-hook abs.

Although genetics play a role in the shape of your musculature, any healthy individual can still achieve their own set of off-the-hook abs.

A skewed vision of abs permeates everywhere we go, even beyond the fitness books, movies and MTV videos. It can't be avoided, even in real life! We often assume that anybody with six-pack abs is in excellent shape, but, believe it or not, this is not necessarily the case. There are individuals out there who are lean and light, with shredded abs, who may not be able to do twenty proper push-ups or a few good pull-ups. That six-pack does not always translate to overall health. However, because of the way our brains have been programmed, we often perceive anyone with excess body fat around the middle (even if they're strong or fit) to be less "in shape" than someone with six-pack abs. I myself am occasionally guilty of this from time to time, so I'll say it again: Although strong abdominal muscles are incredibly important—you literally use them every single time you lift, twist and even stand up—having a six-pack doesn't always guarantee that an individual is fit. It's true there is a gigantic overlap, but I'd consider it more of a correlation than direct result.

Ironically, the fact that ripped, shredded abs do not 100% guarantee absolute power and functional strength has caused a small backlash within select fitness circles. I have personally heard both trainers and fitness enthusiasts whom I respect in others ways, berate the notion of training specifically for abs. I however believe there's a time and place for just about everything in this universe of health. Why put down anything that makes people thoughtful about nutrition and happier with themselves?

In fact, just about everyone who ever trained hard has at some point focused on abs for *aesthetic* purposes. Even you cavemen, cavewomen and functional fitness fanatics out there have to admit that *somewhere along the line,* maybe twenty years ago or more, you did do sit-ups for looks. Perhaps leg raises or even crunches; *something* to target those abs.

Let's be honest. It's important in fitness and life.

Further, we must be honest about working hard. Some of us claim to have met someone along the way who "eats whatever they want" and "doesn't work out," yet still has excellent abs. If you truly have met someone as such, then I will not argue with you. But I will point out that such an individual is extremely rare. Most of us have to earn it.

Results will come with hard work and time, but it's usually not a straight path.

When I say "earn it", I mean that you must make sacrifices. You will have to implement dietary adjustments. Although I do not advise obsessive calorie counting or keeping a food journal, you will have to be more aware than ever of what, and how much, you eat. This is not easy. You will also have to train 'til your body aches, consistently and intensely, again and again. Luckily, I enjoy hard work. I feel that most people on the path to fitness do as well. So please do not see "earn it" as a deterrent. It *feels good* to earn something!

There will be times where me must exercise restraint. I do not advocate deprivation, but we must be realistic. In other words, you can have an ice cream cone some of the time, you just can't have every single ice cream cone all of the time. Again, it comes down to honesty. It's incredible how often we kid ourselves about the quantities we eat and drink. Although we will discuss nutrition more extensively in Part II, I'd like to be perfectly clear here and now: It is impossible to acquire the lean, shredded six-pack of your dreams without being realistic and aware of what and how much you're putting in your body. Like I often say, what you eat is probably the single most important decision you can make in your journey.

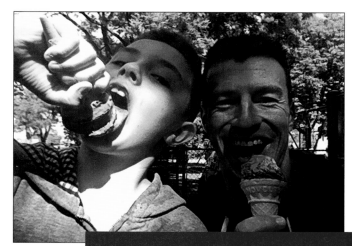

You can have an ice cream cone some of the time, you just can't have every single ice cream cone all of the time.

There is an alarming lack of honesty in the diet and fitness industry. I am certainly not the first to make this assertion. It can seem as though everybody from the gym, to the trainers, to the supplement companies, to the equipment manufacturers want to tell you that their way is the best, that it's guaranteed to work for you and everyone else—yeah, right!

In life and fitness, there are no guarantees.

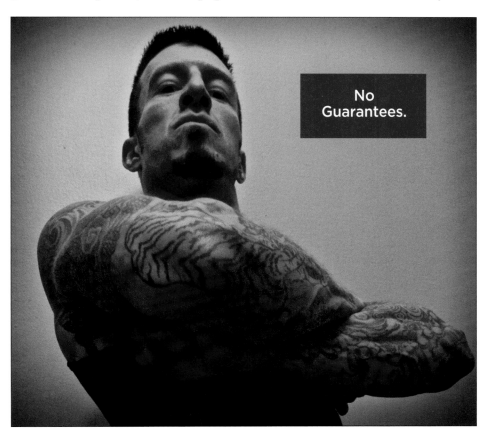

No Guarantees.

This book contains everything you need to know about sculpting and maintaining amazing, defined and beautiful abs. I pored over every detail to provide as much useful information as I could for every exercise, dietary and lifestyle recommendation in these pages. But you have to do all the work. That's right, all of it. I'll give you the tools, but you do everything. This book does not guarantee a six-pack. It doesn't guarantee anything. Enjoy it! There is nothing more empowering than using your own physical and mental effort to change. If this book helps you, then HELLYEAH!

> An abs program should be supplemental to, not in place of, a full body program. Squatting, Pushing and Pulling are still essential.

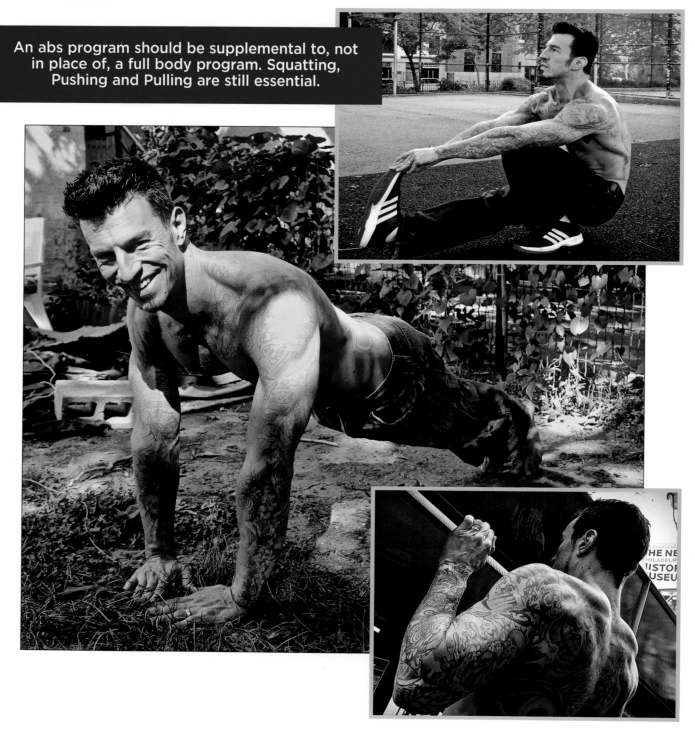

The abs programs and exercises detailed herein are intended to be part of your over-all fitness protocol. Yes, you still must train legs; you still need to train your whole body. Squatting, pushing and pulling are essential when we train. Don't worry; they're good for abs too.

Even before I worked as a professional fitness trainer, people asked me about abs all the time. Of course now, it's more than ever--even more so than calisthenics or tattoos. "How do you get abs?" folks inquire, as if there is something I did or said once in the past rendering my abs chiseled in the present. Or maybe I half-stepped my way through an easy work-out every now and again. Sometimes that's what people want to hear. You can't fault them: it's what they're used to hearing from others, but they'll never hear it from me.

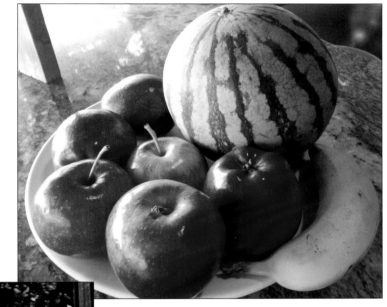

I recommend that one eat well and train hard, frequently and consistently, for a prolonged, undetermined duration, hopefully for life. It's an even playing field, but it's not going to happen on it's own and it's not going to happen overnight. You and only you are accountable.

One more thing as long as we're being 100% honest: No equipment is needed to get your abs (or the rest of your body) into the best shape of your life. That's right, none whatsoever. Although some of the exercises contained herein make use of minimalist gear (like a bar for instance), all you need to get the ultimate Diamond-Cut six-pack of your dreams is you!

No equipment is necessary.

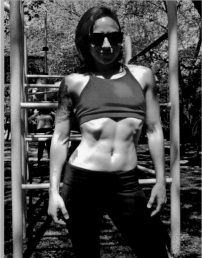

All races, age groups, genders, social classes, sexual orientations, and walks of life are into abs. Love it or hate it, the obsession with abs is a cultural phenomenon that transcends culture. And it ain't goin' anywhere!

Diamond-Cut Abs come in all shapes and sizes.

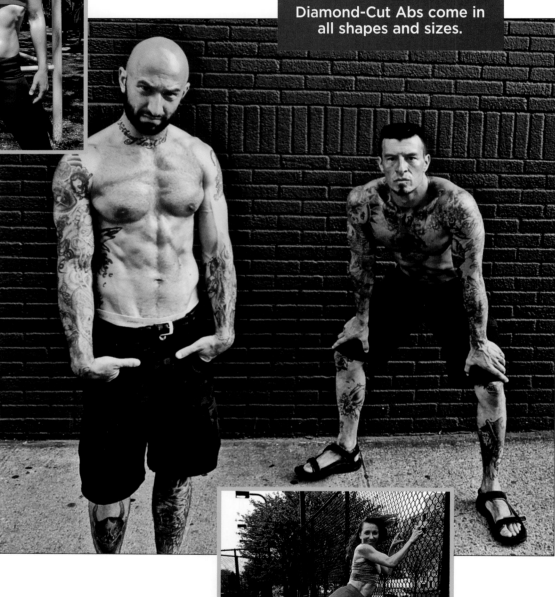

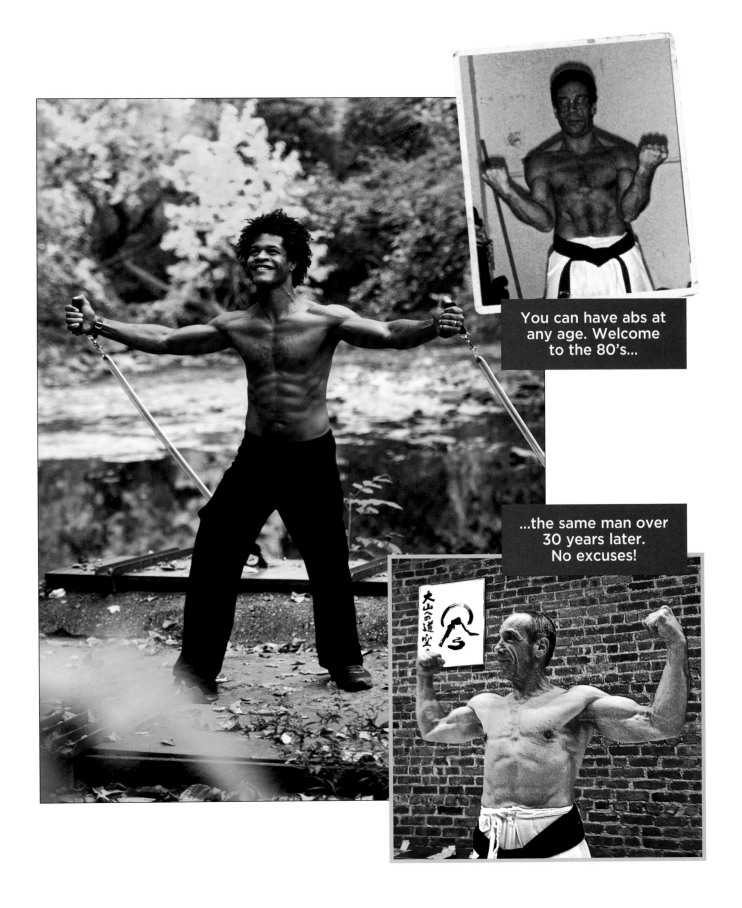

You can have abs at any age. Welcome to the 80's...

...the same man over 30 years later. No excuses!

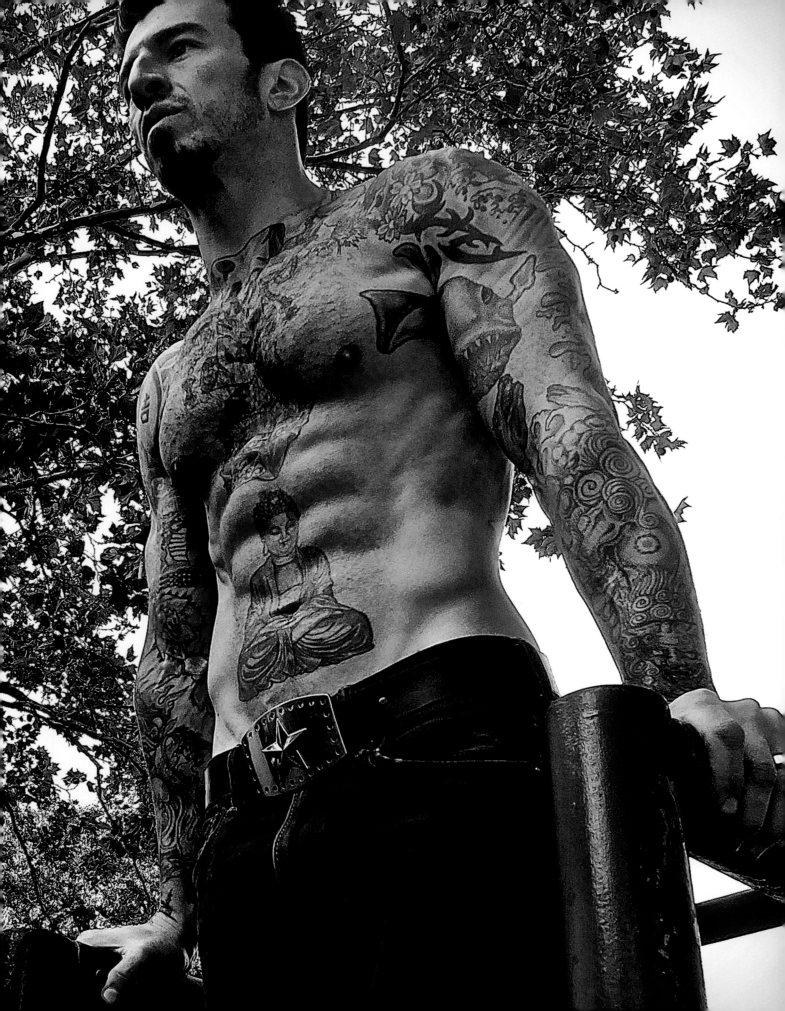

CHAPTER 2

ABS DEFINED

Almost everything in our world is expected to happen instantly. If it takes thirty-five minutes to get a pizza, we flip out. If it takes thirty-five seconds for the internet to connect, then we raise Holy Hell! When I was a kid, the invention of "One-Hour Photo" was unbelievably fast. But it would be interminably slow by today's standard of "Right Now Photo". It is easy to get swept up and forget that, as technology has changed, our bodies have not. So, while we are constantly bombarded with images of speedy metamorphoses, 7-minute abs and 21-day transformations, we must accept that these things are false, despite how much they can seem real.

Marketing is marketing. Much of the time, the images of transformations are brought to you by someone trying to sell you something. To make the sale, they can and will make it look like whatever they want it to. You can shoot dramatic before and after pictures five minutes apart. This should be obvious in the modern era, but sometimes we don't realize it. After all, the Man is very good at pulling the proverbial wool over our eyes. Hell, if the medium of visual technology can make it look like Will Smith is saving the world from aliens or that Elijah Wood is a hobbit, then it can certainly give the illusion of unrealistically speedy transformations.

Never forget, no matter what anyone says, you cannot fake the funk. Changing your body requires time, persistence, hard work and patience. It's very rare for change manifest quickly. If incorporated in your life, the efforts and adjustments required for a ripped set of abs are not a big deal. Most people spend more time on facebook or playing Candy Crush than I do working on my abs, but I'm consistent and intense. In fitness you truly reap what you sow. If you make effort, it shows. That's the beauty of it. Many things worth doing do not come easy.

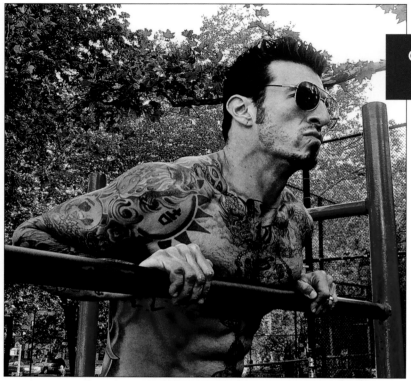

Get over it! Many things worth doing do not come easy.

So, as we know, the magazines, ads and movies are not rooted in reality, but what is? Pardon the pun, but how do we literally *define* abs?

When we talk about "abs" we are referring to a general part of the body (the anterior mid-section), as well as several specific muscles. Please be warned that I am about to be uncharacteristically technical for a brief moment. Forgive me; this is as academic as I get. Here are the muscles:

First is the *rectus abdominis*. This is the "six-pack" of legend. In reality, it is only one muscle that runs vertically over the whole abs area, from the pubic bone all the way up to the chest. The tendinous intersections can give it the look of six or even eight separate cubes, depending on genetics and other factors. The rectus abdominis pulls the sternum and hips toward each other, and is responsible for tilting the pelvis.

Next is the *transverse abdominal*. It spans horizontally across the abdominal wall and is the deepest of the abs muscles. The transverse abdominal pulls the abs inward, like a vacuum, expelling air.

Obliques are responsible for trunk rotation, and run diagonally. They are the "side" muscles. There are two types, each with a right and left counterpart. The internal obliques twist the trunk to the same side. (The left one is activated when twisting to the left.) The external obliques twist toward the opposite side. (The left one is activated when twist to the *right*.)

The *serratus anterior* would not make most lists, as it is technically not an abdominal muscle, but I would not think of omitting it. The portion of the serratus anterior that is visible form the front is a huge part of the ultimate abs look. It frames and shapes the six-pack and can make or break the upper body's overall appearance. The serratus anterior lifts, abducts and rotates the scapula (shoulder blades). Bar-work (and thus, all hanging abs) are phenomenal for it.

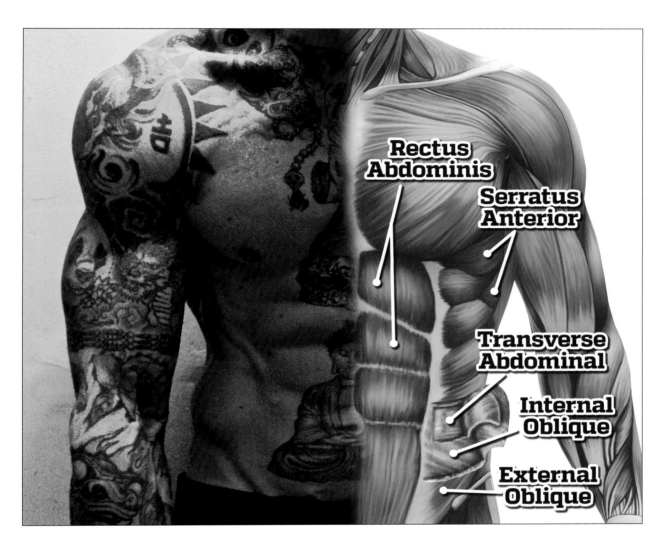

In abdominal training, the phrases "upper abs" and "lower abs" are often used. While we know that the rectus abdominis is one single muscle, it is undeniable that certain exercises target higher or lower, emphasizing certain areas more than others. Furthermore, the tendons running across practically provide a visual diagram for "upper" and "lower". Although potentially anatomically misleading, the use of these terms can be helpful for beginners when trying to zone in on an exercise. Naturally, I believe that the whole body functions cohesively. It's a huge part of my overall approach to fitness and something I treasure about body-weight training. (More on this in Part III.)

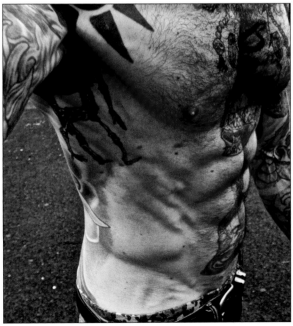

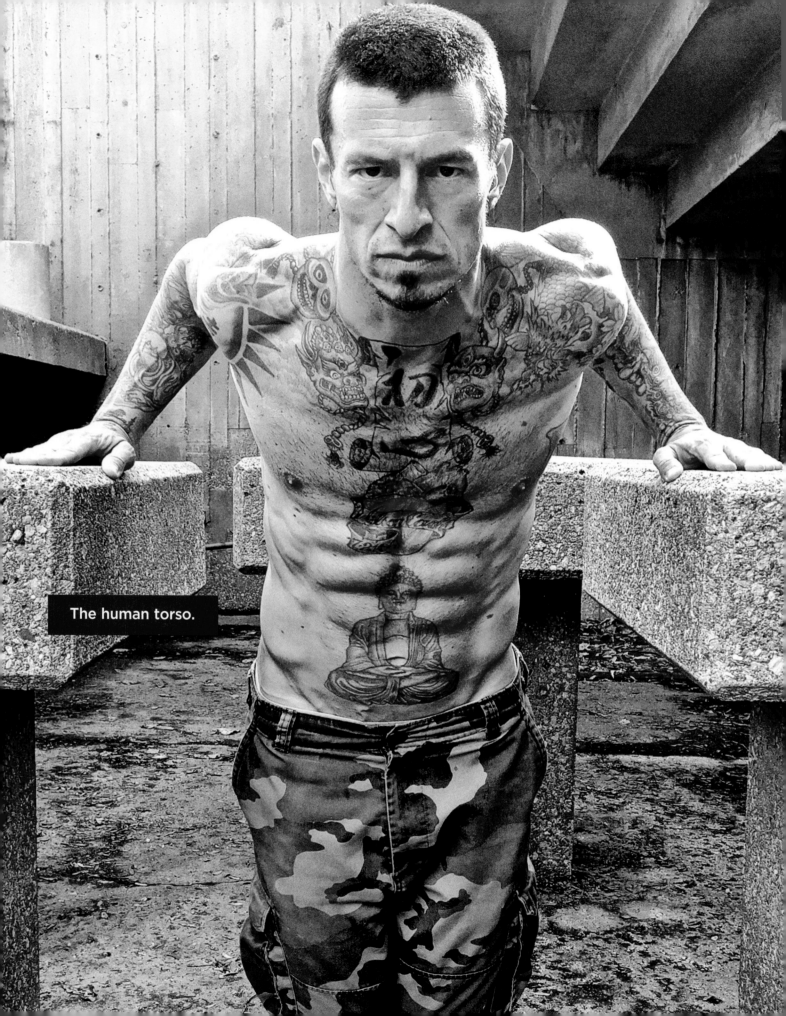

The human torso.

"Core" is another term that gets thrown around a lot. Merriam-Webster's dictionary defines it as "a central and often foundational part". Indeed. In the exercise kingdom, "core" is somewhat subjective, open to interpretation. I consider the core to include the entire human torso: chest, back, shoulders, butt, hip flexors, spine erectors and, of course, abs. Although this book is about "abs", not about "core", we don't have to get hung up on semantics—they're just words, baby. The body is the body.

I believe that there is no true separation or isolation in the first place. If I am an ocean then my every muscle, bone and fiber is a drop of water. I cannot really distinguish. As Bruce Lee said, "Be water, my friend."

There are many benefits to having a strong core / abdominal area / mid-section / "powerhouse". (I don't like to get hung up on semantics.) They include increased strength, improved posture and balance, faster metabolism, better performance and fewer aches and pains, to name just a few.

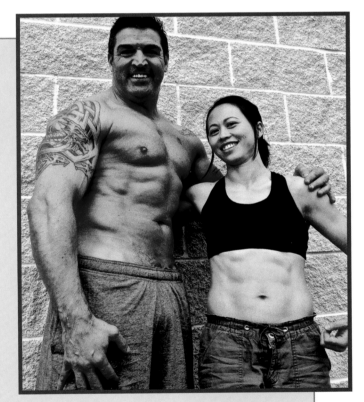

On Genetics

The shape of every body part is dictated by genetics. It's why some people are taller than others and why your nose is shaped differently than mine. So why is it so hard to understand that our abs can be different sizes and shapes too? My square abs cannot be round any more than my size 13 feet can be 10. But like your abs, or the abs of any healthy, uninjured individual, they have the potential to be out of this world!

Whatever the distinctions of your personal musculature, you are still capable of earning ultimate, Diamond-Cut Abs. A lifter and a gymnast would tend to have different genetic traits, but both are amazingly fit. It's the same thing with anybody's different looking abs. Any healthy person can be ripped, toned and carved out of wood, even if we look different. No exceptions.

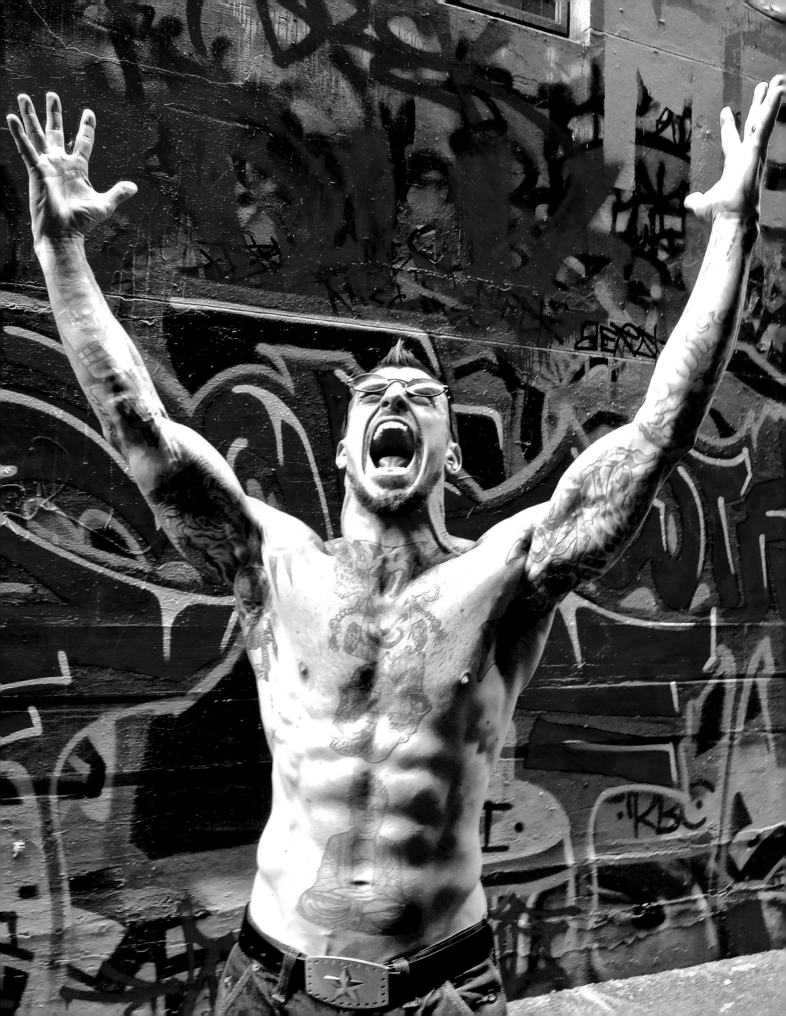

CHAPTER 3

PERSONAL OBSESSION

I was born in Brooklyn, New York, the scorching summer of '74 in a hospital currently in a battle just to stay open. It's almost symbolic to me, a sign of the times. A lot has changed. Things come and go, I suppose. Without trying to play sociologist, I will simply say that the Brooklyn youth of that era had a certain edge that I fear will be lacking in future generations.

In the seventies, eighties, and even the nineties, there was an unspoken "tough guy" element intrinsically wired in anyone who grew up here and survived. Even though the streets were a thousand times rougher then, our generation played outside. We were streetwise. We witnessed the birth of rap and the numerous "deaths" of rock. Over the years, my generation of Brooklynites experienced the rise of everything from *Saturday Night Fever*, to Biggie Smalls, to Biohazard and everything in between. Culturally speaking there will never be anything like it again. The internet may as well have been ten thousand years away. We didn't even have cable TV in my neighborhood; we had UHF. Everything had to be seen as it happened. Brooklyn was the world's biggest small town.

No, this isn't San Quentin. It's the schoolyard at Bildersee Junior High. I was in the class of '87.

I had a nonathletic upbringing and was discouraged from participating in sports as a youth. My psychotic gym teacher reinforced this. All I remember about elementary school gym class is getting screamed at. I recall feeling unsettled and angry. Once in a while, we played dodgeball and, if we were lucky, did some jumping jacks and sit-ups. This was the early 80's, so the sit-ups were old school, full range of motion—the kind that, years later, some decried as "bad for you". Sit-ups were the first abs exercise that I, and so many others from my generation, ever did.

I liked sit-ups but hated gym.

In spite of this burning hatred, somehow, my brothers and I discovered strength training at a young age. Looking back, I honestly don't know how it happened. It must have been a combination of watching local hero Lou Ferrigno on *The Incredible Hulk*, along with our own God-given testosterone (not to mention the competitive nature of a household with three boys). The desire to not get our asses kicked at school probably played a role too. It's hard to say exactly.

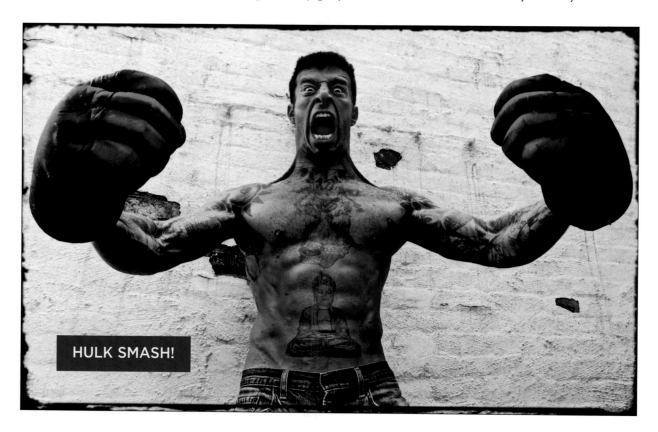

HULK SMASH!

I think we fell specifically into body weight training early on because, aside from a dusty piece of pipe for pull-ups, we couldn't afford equipment. I was young when I did my first push-ups and pull-ups, and I'm grateful for that. I did those two exercises non-stop, as I still do to this very day. I maintain that push-ups and pull-ups gave me an unbelievable strong foundation for abs and so much more, on which I would build later in life, as my obsession bloomed. No equipment needed but the bar!

Like most boys, eventually I wanted to grow so I acquired a used bench and some dumbbells. I started lifting as a teenager, when I discovered girls. I generally stuck to the classic "Brooklyn Workout": chest & tri's twice a week, back & bi's twice a week, shoulders once, abs all days. It was all about taking my shirt off and back then. Legs were regretfully lacking in my youthful ignorance; such was the style at the time.

Although I switched to a "split-routine" when I got the weights (a training style which I've since switched back out of), no matter what body part I trained, I always did abs too. At this point I had expanded beyond the sit-up and was messing around with declines and transverse motions like crossovers. Although I was lean and getting undeniably stronger and more muscular, my abs were not progressing at a rate that I found acceptable, nor did they have anywhere close to the appearance I was striving for. Many of us have experienced this type of frustration in our training.

Soon I found out about leg raises. I started doing extra obliques exercises. "Aha!" I thought. "Time to step up my game! More is more!" I believed, like many others at the time, that increasing my reps would automatically yield lean, shredded abs. I also got involved in nutrition and started cooking most of my meals, growing more aware of the effects of food on my physiology. This probably did far more for my abs than the rep increase did.

I made a decision to have ultimate, Diamond-Cut Abs.

At nineteen years of age, I started training abs a minimum of five days a week. I did three hundred reps every single session… minimum. This was probably the peak of my obsession with abs. This "peak" lasted over ten years, although these days, I have a *very* different approach and do a lot fewer reps! Ironically my abs are both functionally stronger and more aesthetically appealing than they were back then, even with *way* fewer reps… but I'm skipping ahead.

In June of 1994, two months shy of my twentieth birthday, I answered an ad in the Village Voice. There was no Craig's List then and people still read papers. The ad said, "Punk band needs drummer for European tour". That's it.

Two weeks later, I was on a plane to Frankfurt, Germany beginning thirty days of rock shows across several countries. I did abs almost every day of that tour, no matter the situation, no kid-

ding. Sometimes it was on the beer-soaked, splintered, wooden floor in the back of some dive; sometimes it was worse. You must understand the extent of my obsession. I spent the night in mad places with crazed people, but always got my three hundred reps. One time, we played a show in the village of Bremervorde and had to stay in an abandoned barn that some punk kids were squatting in. I was supposed to sleep on a mattress that wreaked so badly of urine and ass that I chose to sleep outside with the chickens instead. Next morning, I did my three hundred reps on a bed of hay and bird droppings. I was *that* committed to the program.

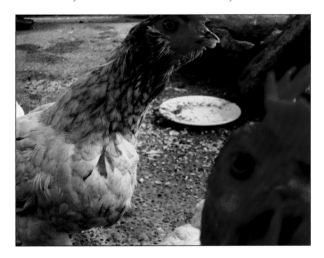

Other nights were more glamorous, but, sometimes even sadly, just as obsessive. A week after the barn incident, we stayed in the city of Nice in Southern France. On our first night, we sat under the stars of the countryside. Our hosts provided us with a truly French dining experience, which I'll never forget.

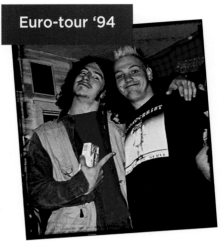

Euro-tour '94

We had the full spread: wine, fruit, breads and, of course, a smoldering pot of fondue. As the delicious aroma filled the air, you could hear the soft, gentle bubbling sound in the background. But this was at a time when I was obsessed with abs and, unfortunately, somewhat misguided. Regretfully, I subscribed to the mid-90's conventional wisdom pertaining to so-called "fat grams". So, in a decision with which I'm still uncomfortable to this day, I declined the fondue. It disgusts me to admit, but it's true. Ugh. Obviously I feel differently now: Cheese is good; counting fat grams is not.

You see, back then I read every book and nutrition label I could get my hands on and, like many others, I found lots of conflicting information. I was young and green and considered everything. Ultimately, I had to experiment for myself. It wasn't until later, when I did my own research about nutrition (i.e. observation and common sense) that I came to reject the notions of both "fat" and "grams" as they pertain to six pack abs—they seem silly and irrelevant. I now put more focus on the quality of real ingredients.

Who was I? A fundamental principle of my life philosophy is I don't believe in regrets: there are things you do and things you don't do. But I'll be damned if I don't regret passing on that fondue. No vanity muscle is worth compromising a new life experience. Deprivation is not healthy. Looking back, I should have partaken in the goodness, which I absolutely would have today. Oh well, at least I drank the wine!

Fast forward a few years: The obsession raged on and I became even more driven.

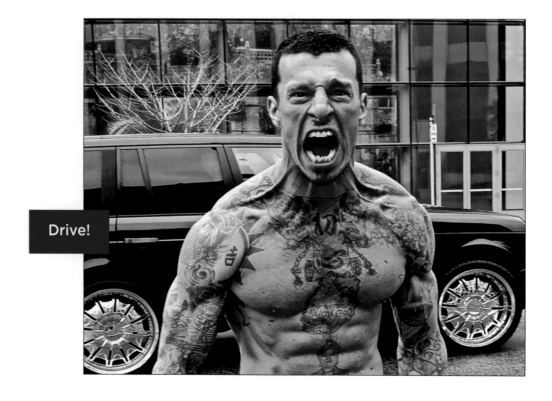

Drive!

I worked in a restaurant in late 90's, shucking clams and delivering food on a broken bicycle in Chelsea. Good times. I woke up before 6am every day, early enough to have my coffee, take a shit, do my abs, take a shower and ride my bike ten miles to work. When I'd get there, I'd have two scoops of creatine powder dissolved in a high-carbohydrate beverage. I currently recommend neither creatine nor high carbohydrate, sugary beverages, but again, I was young and experimenting. It's amazing how, looking back, I believed so much hype. Part of my mission in this book is to help distinguish the bullshit from the truth. Although I fancied myself a free thinker and had enough sense to question authority, drop out of college, and run to Europe in a band (part of how I wound up a grown-up delivery guy, but that's another story), I still had to learn the hard way, the only way: experience.

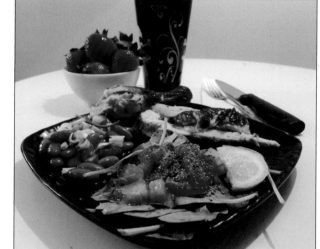

An amateur body-builder named J worked in the kitchen. As a student himself of physical culture, he was sensitive to my eating habits. Instead of the cheap grease and sugar-laden, chicken-fried staff meals that the other employees gorged on, J would cook me chicken, beans and a green salad every day, sometimes with strawberries for dessert. I still eat that same meal several times a week. It's one of my favorites.

In those days, I hit the gym about five days a week. I started drinking protein shakes around this time too. I bought into the lie of protein shakes for longer than I care to admit. It was one of the last fallacies I was able to do away with. My abs and every single other part of me, including my digestive system, are better than ever since eliminating protein supplements.

I believed in creatine and protein powders at the time, just like I believed that fat grams mattered more than actual food. Yes creatine makes your muscles swole with water, but it does little else. Yes, muscular growth requires protein—they are the "building blocks" after all, but the processed powder is garbage, even if the label says "high quality." I am a firm believer that you can build lean, strong muscle with nothing more than the food you eat and the way you train. Getting world-class washboard abs requires no supplements at all.

I still train my ass off but my approach to exercise is different than it was back then. In my current training style, I focus less on repetition and more on the quality of movement. I'm less goal-oriented and more process-oriented. At this stage, I am proud of where my abs and I are, but I am still growing, looking to learn more and be further challenged. To finish means to be through with it. I'm just getting started.

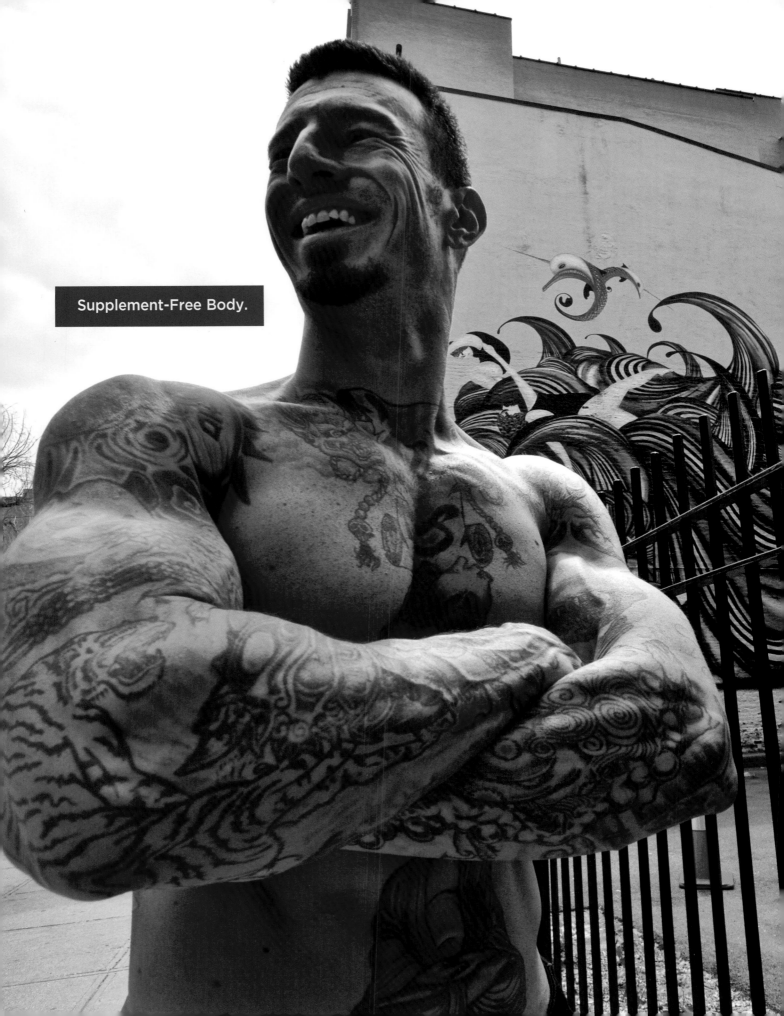

Supplement-Free Body.

"To finish a work? To finish a picture? What nonsense!
To finish it means to be through with it."
–Pablo Picasso

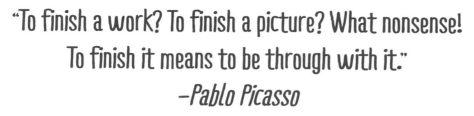

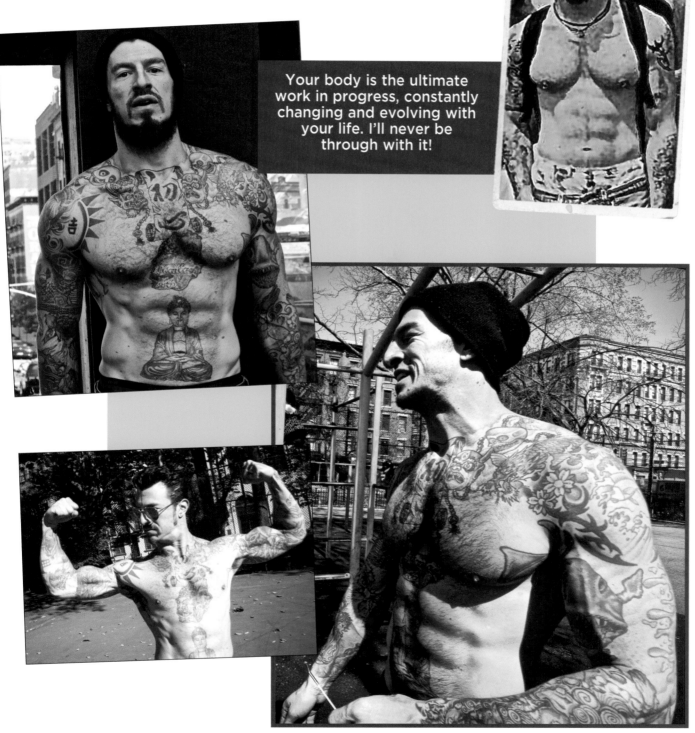

Your body is the ultimate work in progress, constantly changing and evolving with your life. I'll never be through with it!

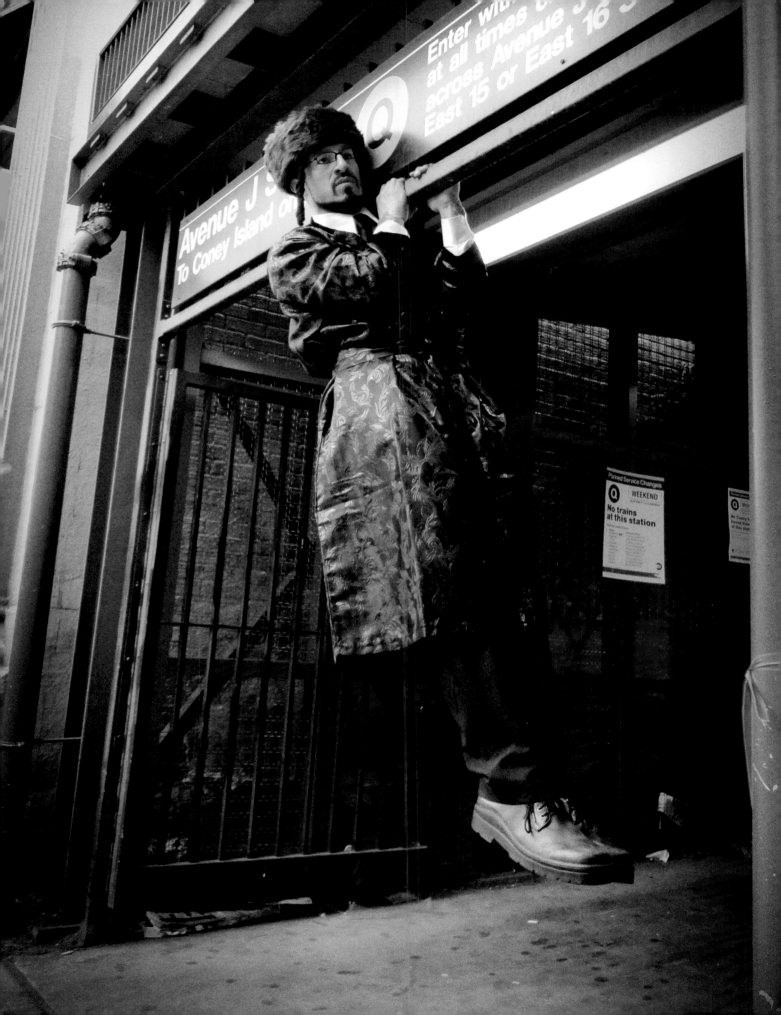

PART II
NUTRITIONAL MUSINGS

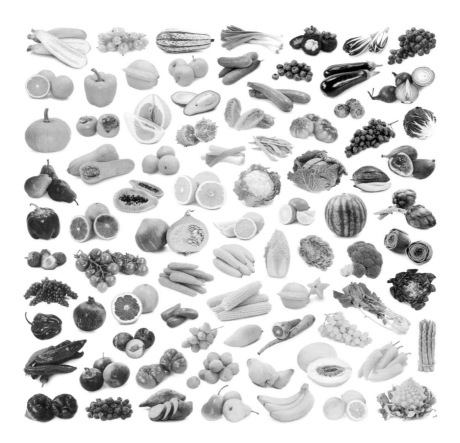

"There can be no joy without food or drink."
—The Talmud

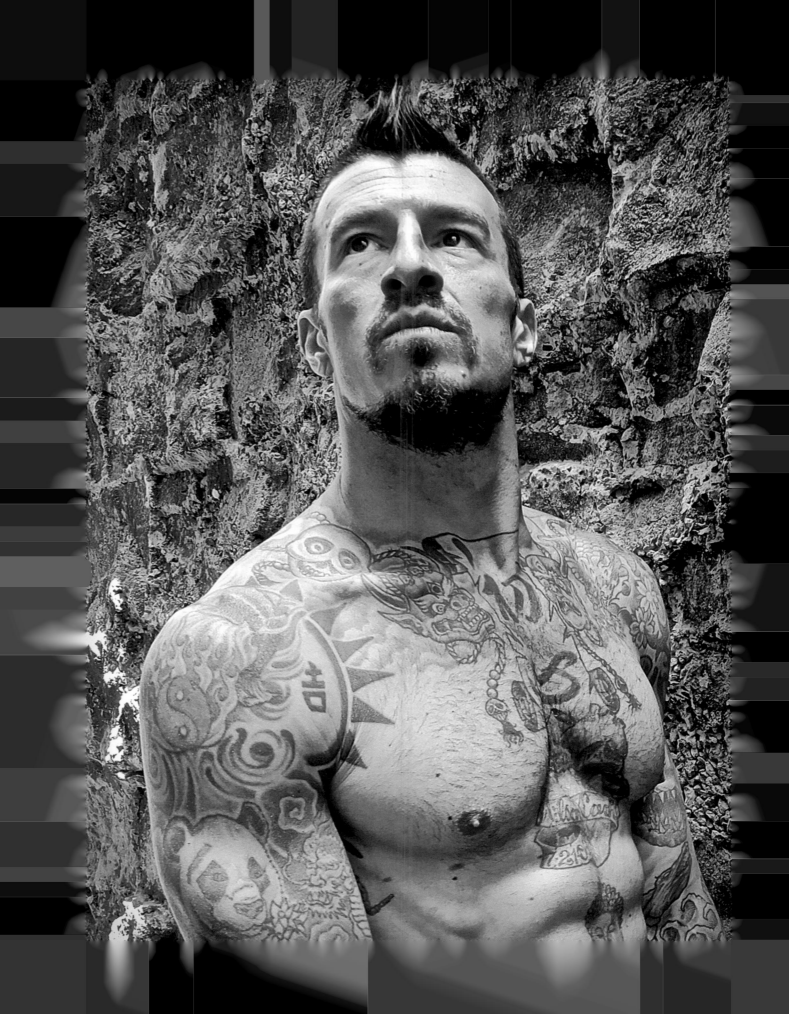

CHAPTER 4

PRIMORDIAL SOUP

E All living things eat. It is as essential as breathing: a physical, biological necessity. No one has to be told to do it. When the earth was a big, molten, swampy ball, the first protozoa who ever spawned (or split in half... I can't recall much from 9th grade biology) knew it must eat or die, even though it lacked a brain and nervous system.

Eating is beyond instinct. A human baby can't do much besides eat, breathe, shit and grab (I consider the latter to be evidence of pull-ups being deep-rooted in our DNA, but that's a separate discussion.)

The digestive system converts food into fuel. Food provides energy to the entire body. No legitimate scientist, theologist, nutritionist, dietician, coach or trainer with any integrity, would ever dispute that *ya' gotta eat to live!*

For advanced creatures like us, however, food plays many roles beyond mere sustenance. We love food.

I love food!

Food provides us with joy. Meals are part of celebrations and holidays. Great moments in life are often marked with food. We cherish family recipes; we reminisce about restaurants we dined at with past lovers; we dream of foods we ate as kids. Comfort food.

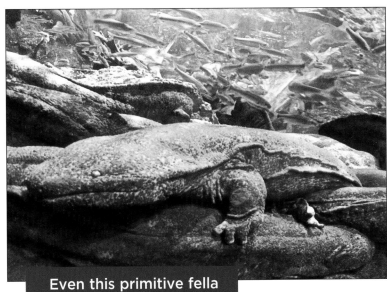

Even this primitive fella knows he's gotta eat.

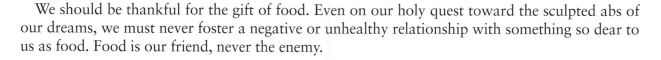

Meals should be enjoyed, prepared and eaten with care.
Sometimes I'm lucky enough to have prepared the food myself!

We have favorite dishes and foods we hate. Whichever the case, we are passionate!

I once attended a New York City fire escape pig roast. I ate freshly caught mahi mahi in Mexico and dined on raw horse sashimi in Tokyo. I shared fermented herring in Sweden and homegrown blood sausage in Ireland with my extended calisthenics family. Food goes beyond taste; it's a spectacular celebration of culture and heritage. Life and joy. Experience.

We should be thankful for the gift of food. Even on our holy quest toward the sculpted abs of our dreams, we must never foster a negative or unhealthy relationship with something so dear to us as food. Food is our friend, never the enemy.

We have risen from the primordial soup, and learned to walk on two legs. We can talk and even cook. We can think, drive and fall in love. But the extent of our love affair with food may be the only thing that truly separates us from the animals.

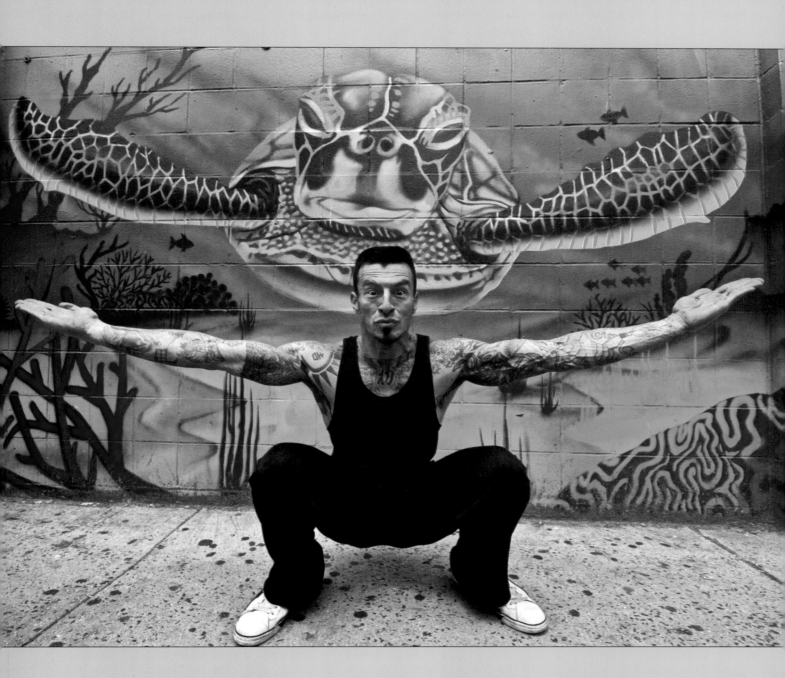

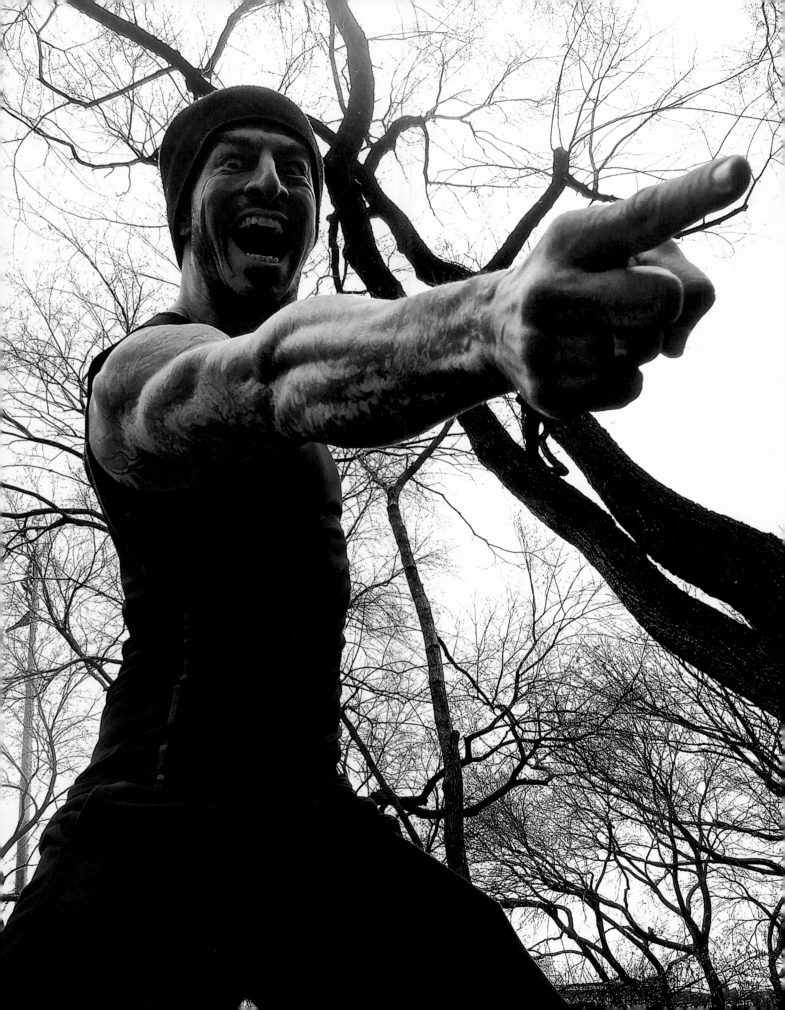

CHAPTER 5

COMMON SENSE VS.
OVER-COMPARTMENTALIZATION

When we're talking about the food we eat, which I believe is the single most important decision we can make regarding our abs, not to mention our overall health, there is a lot of madness to sift through. We are told many conflicting accounts from various sources. It can be hard to know what decisions to make. Ultimately, you and only you are accountable for your choices. Experiment with my advice, but do not to take it as gospel. Find what works for you. This is only my experience.

That said, let's drop any preconceived notions and keep an open mind. Tread lightly... what you are about to read may not be what you're used to hearing.

First things first: I am not a registered dietician. I do not have a college education and I tend to reject most conventional wisdom when it comes to matters of nutrition. I consider the teachings of the few "sports nutrition" and "weight loss specialist" certifications that I possess to be total BS like all too many certificates and "credits" in fitness, school and life.

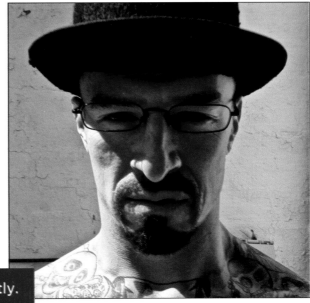

Tread lightly.

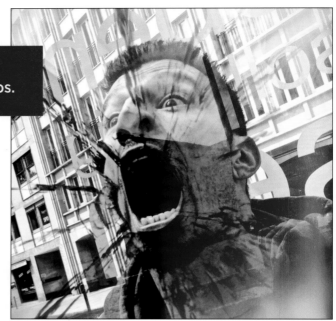

NOOO!!! There's not a correlation between academic credentials and abs.

My textbook credentials may *appear* misleading to those who are into paperwork, yet lots of people pay me for my nutritional advice. Technically, I am a nutritionist (of which there is no official definition, unlike RD—*Registered Dietician*—which has specific, legal requirements). Despite having so few letters after my name, my abs are shredded! Even more so than the bellies of any RD's I've ever met. How is that possible? Somehow I achieved a great set of abs without even knowing what a ketone was.

There is no correlation between a person's academic accomplishments and their abs. How else can you explain the co-existence of soft doctors and sculpted athletes who, perhaps, have not gone to college to study organic chemistry, epidemiology or other such pre-med requirements? I've known lots of guys who haven't even completed high school, but I'd take their nutritional guidance over that of an ample-bodied dietician or portly coach any day. Experience over education. Lots of people I trust are not fitness professionals, but they use a "common sense" approach to nutrition. Practical over theoretical.

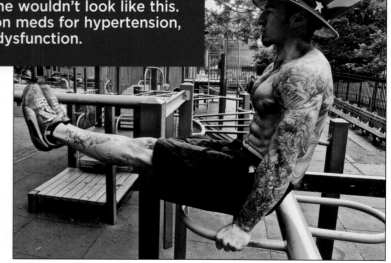

Sadly, the USDA is on the take when it comes to nutritional guidance. If Uncle Sam were real, he wouldn't look like this. He'd be obese and take prescription meds for hypertension, anxiety and erectile dysfunction.

Personally, I am someone who has studied the effects of exercise and eating styles firsthand, through over 25 years of training and dietary experimentation with myself, as well as with many clients and peers. We see what works. Defenders of the Status Quo might advise against my teachings. They may say to trust the USDA, with their corrupt food pyramid and recommendations of non-stop processed grains. But I say to observe what's in front of you. The fat cats are not the ones to believe--only your eyes. When you employ the methods detailed herein, it is likely you will both enjoy every meal more *and* look better with your shirt off.

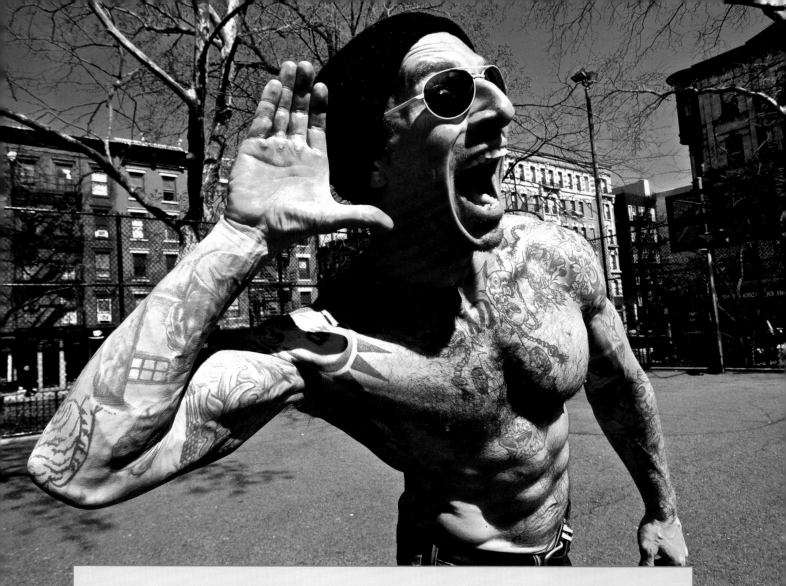

Hear Me Out

I would like to happily acknowledge the fact that others have gotten results with methods other than mine. I applaud them for it! However, I will only discuss what I've personally seen work. The dietary guidance expressed in this section has proven effective for me and 100% of the people I've known to actually embrace it. Again, that figure is 100%. Hear me out.

Fit humans have existed way before the invention/discovery/nomenclature of nutrition. I believe that optimum abs can be attained without thinking too much about the labels or components of food at all. That's precisely what I'm referring to when I talk about over-compartmentalization— the practice of focusing on food parts and nutritional variables, rather than on the *foods themselves*. The whole is always greater than the sum of its parts.

In efforts to categorize and understand things, nutritional science has invented the classifications of macro-nutrients (fats, carbohydrates, proteins) and micro-nutrients (vitamins, minerals). More recently, science has "discovered" (huh?) what has come to be known as anti-oxidants.

And guess what… They have existed in real food all along! No one will ever understand why a strawberry is so special. We can spend years analyzing it in a laboratory, but we'll never know. What is it about a scallion or a Brussels spout that's so complex, delicious and perfect?

Who cares?

All too often, we confuse "complicated" or "time consuming" with "important". In realty there is not usually a correlation. Each food is extraordinary for what it is. Kinda' like people.

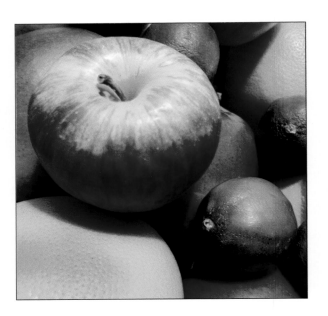

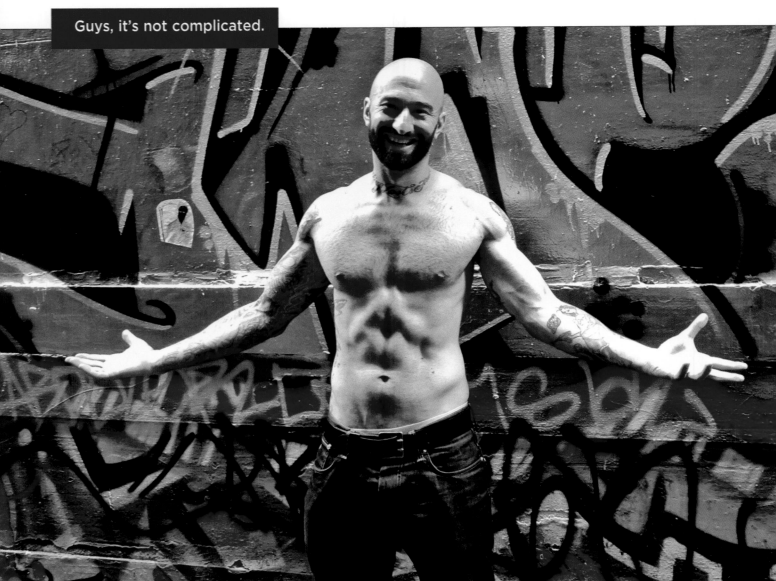

Guys, it's not complicated.

Master Of Reality

When I talk about" real", I am referring to fruits, vegetables, nuts, legumes and seeds. The closer they are to nature, the better. Meaning, a peach is real and a jar of preserved, sugared peaches is not.

I also consider animal products like fish, red meat, eggs and dairy to be "real". Like the aforementioned peach, a farm raised T-bone is real. A Whopper Jr. is not.

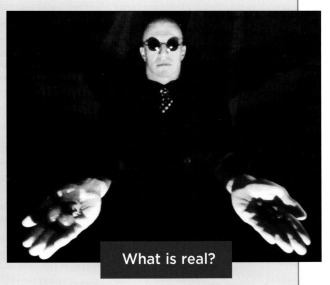

What is real?

When it comes to foods with ingredients, less is more. Generally, I consider homemade breads and pastas to be "real", as they don't contain much more than water, flour, salt and yeast. Conversely, there are many chemicals and preservatives found in most commercial wheat products on your grocers' shelves. Look at the ingredients. What you find might surprise you.

The decision to eat meat, dairy, grains or whatever is a personal one. Whatever you choose, keep it close to the source whenever possible. Most packaged, processed or chemically enhanced foods are not included in my description, although, sadly, they are sometimes difficult to avoid. But not impossible.

Folks like me prefer not to pay much mind to fat grams and the like, and approach what we eat in terms of "fruit", "meat", "milk", "greens", etc. My type of thinking encourages one to look at colors and prepare meals, rather than look at labels and do math. The latter distances us from what we really need, and what we're really eating. Over-compartmentalization of nutrition promotes ass-backwards thinking—in a quest for ultimate abs, we start choosing foods that *claim* to be "low fat" instead of thinking about foods that are low fat, or even better, not thinking about "fat" at all—just flavor, vitality and quality. The fats found in real foods tend to be good. The fats found in fake foods do not. Again, it's better to think about the food than the fat.

Anyone who has visited a commercial supermarket has seen processed desserts that claimed to be "fat free" on the package. Hoards of brainwashed consumers gorge themselves on this stuff, more concerned with hypothetical "fat" than real "dessert". People want to think that they can lose weight by eating cookies. Do we live in Bizarro world? I guarantee no one ever got shredded abs on a cookie diet.

The truth is that most "fat free" or "low fat" items more than make up for any potential benefits normally associated with these boasts by adding sugar, corn syrup, glycerin, emulsifiers and preservatives. They do more harm than good.

Even when my abs are in peak condition, as they are for many of the images in this book, I do not avoid fats. Ever. When I try to get as lean as possible, nuts and nut butters, avocados, and red meat remain staples in my diet. So do butter and olive oil. I eat quality fats liberally and pay them no mind. Natural, quality fats are good. Cheap grease, like the kind in fast food, is not.

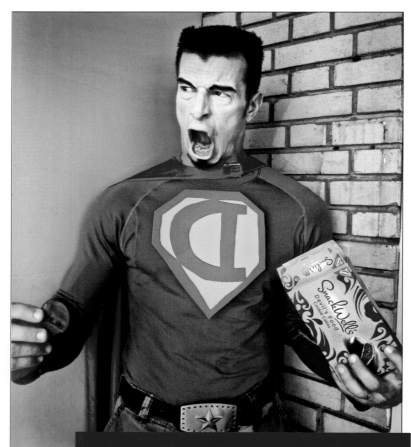

People want to think that they can lose weight by eating "low fat" cookies. Do we live in Bizarro world?

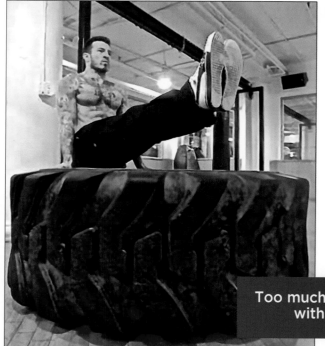

Too much sugar will leave you with a "Spare Tire".

The claim "no high fructose corn syrup" is right up there with "fat free". Often "No HFC" products list "natural cane sugar", "beet sugar" or any number of "nectars" as ingredients. But, in terms of your abs, there is really no distinction. Although the names are less menacing than HFC and they appear to have earthier roots, all these sugars are processed. They all get stored as fat, when not metabolized quickly for energy, often resulting in a "muffin top" or "spare tire".

Gourmet Product?

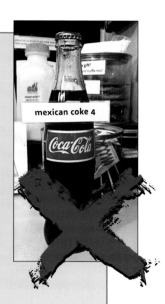

It blew my mind recently when I stepped into a high-end restaurant and saw them selling "Mexican" Coke like it was a gourmet product. (It certainly had a gourmet price tag, considering it's some of the crappiest stuff on Earth.) When I inquired about it, the hostess boasted that in Mexico, Coke is made with real cane sugar! Yes, I am against modified corn products being present in so many food and beverage products, but c'mon! Soda will still make you bloated and gassy no matter what type of pure sugar is in it. It is unlikely you will get abs drinking Coca-Cola in any fashion. Besides, didn't Mexico just surpass the United States as the most overweight nation? Be leery of health claims.

"...Free"

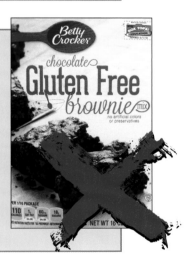

Food products that make health claims should be avoided. Like "sugar free" and "fat free", substances that boast "gluten free" are still often filled with other chemical ingredients. In this case, alkali, soy lecithin and xanthum gum, in addition to the processed sugars and starches that are to be expected. The additives are just as bad for us as gluten, and in many cases, worse. A gluten-free brownie is still a brownie and will not help you get abs. Defer to your own reason and common sense rather that the sales and marketing departments of Betty Crocker.

It's really common sense. Anything made of any type of pure sugar is a hindrance in engineering of the ultimate six-pack. Even unprocessed sugars like raw honey (which does indeed have health benefits) is still pure sugar and can therefore pose a hindrance if you have too much. You cannot get Diamond-Cut Abs if refined sugar is a consistent part of your diet, in anything but a limited capacity. For the record, cane sugar, honey and agave nectar can be just as detrimental to your abs as high fructose corn syrup.

Sugar is one of your abs's greatest enemies. Many people would be surprised to see just how much sugar they consume in a given day if they took an honest look. We all know that soda and candy are pure sugar. But we often do not consider sports drinks, flavored waters, coffee-influenced beverages, energy drinks—many of which make sketchy health claims, but can actually lead to weight gain. Most commercial peanut butter, even "natural style" contains added sugar and is candy. Real natural peanut butter doesn't have more than two ingredients: peanuts and, possibly, salt—no sugar, no palm oil. Sauces, dressings and condiments are usually laden thick with gratuitous sugar. The ignorant and under-informed consume these products freely. To me, one of the biggest issues is that sugar (whether it's called "cane juice" or "corn syrup") is added to products that really have no business containing it in the first place. Items like canned tomatoes, soups and even water have sugar added to them. It's disgusting.

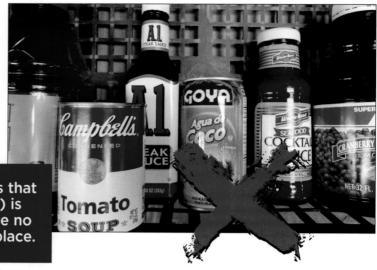

> To me, one of the biggest issues is that sugar (HFC or cane or whatever) is added to products that really have no business containing it in the first place.

I am often asked if I eat a "low carb diet". In truth, I prefer not to think in terms of "low", "carb" or "diet". It's just food! Diets are restrictive by nature. They are meant to be short term. The way I eat is the way I eat. For the most part, I eat minimally prepped and processed foods and I cook a lot. When I eat out, I go to places that use real ingredients. I've eaten this way for years. I stay away from sugar most of the time. I eat plants and animals, cooked with care, and with as few ingredients as possible. Although I don't think much about carbohydrates, when I actually surveyed what I eat in preparation for this chapter, it was revealed that about a third of the foods I eat are indeed carbohydrates— fruits, vegetables, legumes, beans, seeds, etc.--just not much bread, rice, pasta and other grain-derived products. I don't avoid them 100% of the time; they are simply not part of my day-to-day lifestyle. But like birthday cake, there is a time and a place. Sure I cut loose for special occasions--just remember, it's not a special occasion if you do it every day.

By my own admission, my relationship with grains is a complicated one. They have found their way in and out of my eating for years.

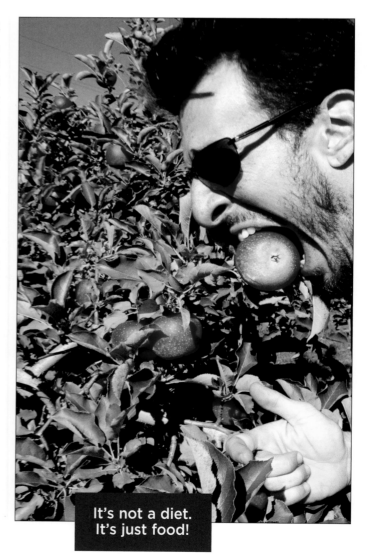

> It's not a diet.
> It's just food!

Truth be told, my abs were at their all time "best" aesthetically a couple of years ago when I went 90 days without any sugar or grain products at all. I ate only meat, fruit, veggies, dairy, legumes and nuts. I also drank plenty of water, and as I recall, a little whiskey. I ate non-stop and got leaner and leaner. Without the sugar and grains, and with a "mostly veggies" eating style, you can eat as much as you want and you will burn your stored body fat for fuel. (It goes without saying that you must train hard.) I strongly believe that the USDA and many other government "experts" advise us to eat way too many grains.

I feel extremely energized when I eat grain-free, at the zenith of metabolic health, but I wholeheartedly acknowledge that not everybody else does. Either way, I don't typically go full-on 100% grain-free for more than a few days a week. Even on days when I do consume grain products, it's far less than what is often recommended, but to each their own. Find what works for you. Going 100% grain and sugar free will shred your abs, and feels great, but for me it is not sustainable every day of my life forever.

Whether grains are 100% good or bad, I cannot say. I do not believe that things are always so black-and-white. To me, the big issue is that Americans are eating grains in disturbingly large amounts. Too much of almost anything will keep you from smashing you abdominal goals, so please be mindful of mow much fuel you're putting in the tank. Additionally, if you do eat bread, you're probably better off getting it from a bakery than a supermarket. Check the list of ingredients if you don't believe me. Commercial bread isn't much better than sugar, even if the package says "whole grain" and has a photo of a brick oven on it. The same is true for rice. Whether it's white or brown, the stuff on the supermarket shelves is all just about the same. Don't believe the hype.

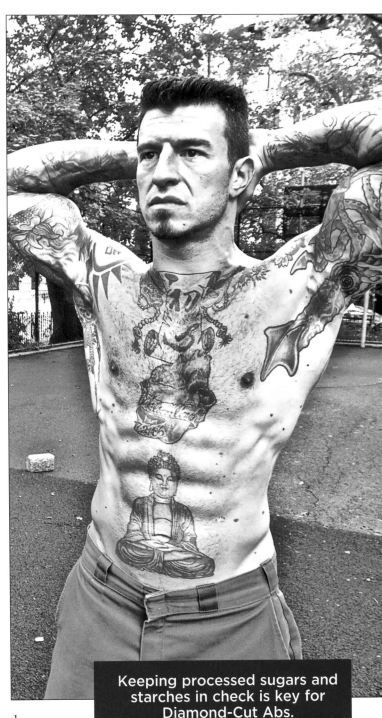

Keeping processed sugars and starches in check is key for Diamond-Cut Abs.

We are surrounded by processed sugar and starch. Keeping them in check is key for getting a shredded six-pack. It has been 100% necessary in my own personal journey toward ultimate abs.

Fruits and vegetables are fantastic. You can feel free to snack on them anytime of day and still maintain extraordinary abs. Fruit is delicious, succulent, sexy and sweet. It blows my mind when I see kids (and grown-ups—*remember, we are in Bizarro World*) snacking on "watermelon" or "grape" artificially flavored treats instead of the real deal. It's madness. Real fruit tastes and feels so good on the tongue. It scratches the itch for something sweet and is packed with life and nutrients. It's as if these folks must have trained their taste buds (and eyes—fruit is gorgeous!) to develop affection for these pretend items. Yes, even the ones made with "Real Fruit" are not fruit. Fruits and veggies have no printed package.

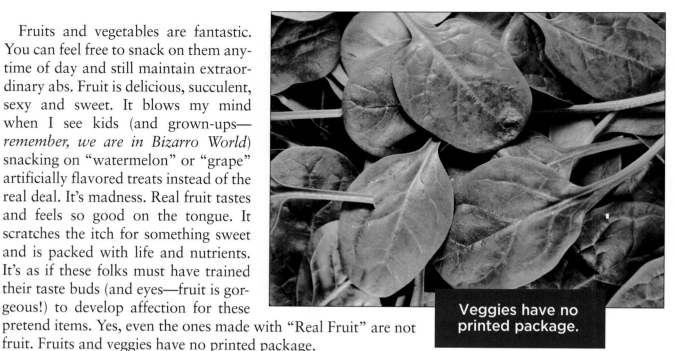

Veggies have no printed package.

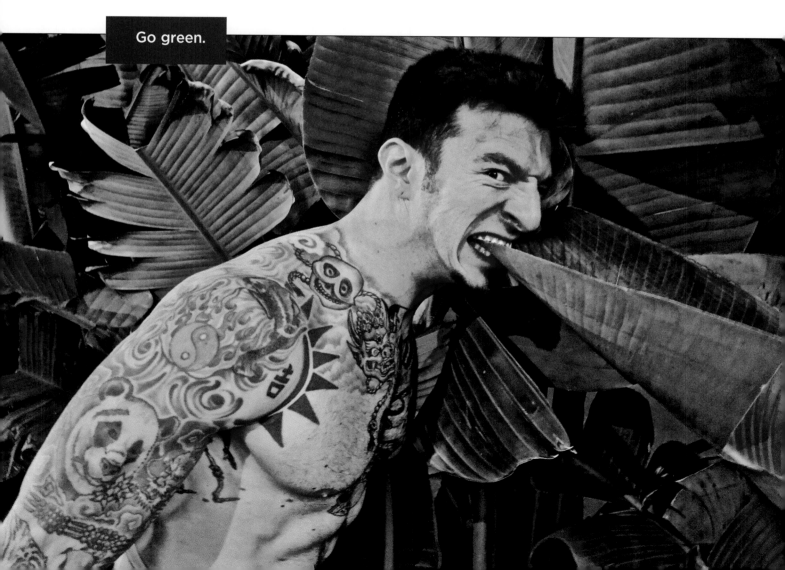

Go green.

Vegetables are spectacular. Enjoy them all day, every day. Eat as many types as you can and cook them as little as possible. They lower the risk of cancer and make your bones strong. Why take a vitamin? Eat your veggies instead. Real food is always better than supplements. In fact, many of the supplements we are encouraged to consume contain artificial versions of the nutrients found in real food, particular leafy greens, herbs and berries. Go directly to the source. Garlic, not garlic pills; fresh berries, not acai powder. Like Michael Pollan says in Food Rules, "Be the kind of person that takes supplements, then skip the supplements." It amazes me how many among us take care to eat clean and then cram fake, processed powders and pills down our filthy feedholes. These products are often more altered and chemically dense than many foods that health-minded consumers go out of their way to avoid. They are not good for you. It's the other healthful habits that lead to wellness, not the stuff in a bottle.

A delicious and practical way to get the vitamins and nutrition your body needs is to eat as many varieties and colors of vegetables and fruits as you can. Red, orange, purple and, of course, green. Lay them out on the counter or table for some visual enticement.

Fruits, veggies and beans are also great sources of fiber. Fiber keeps the metabolism moving and the body regulated. No one's abs look their best when their intestines are backed up. Additionally, the high fiber content helps to enable the nutrients to be absorbed steadily over time, efficiently and effectively, rendering more bang for their buck. This is why eating an apple will always be more conducive to abs than drinking apple juice. When you drink fruit juice, all the good stuff has been removed. It's just sugar, without the fiber. Fruit gives you abs. Fruit juice does not.

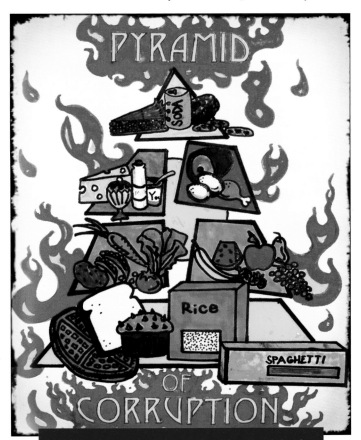

The Food Pyramid (or Pyramid of Corruption, as I like to call it) is a commercial for the government-subsidized refined grain and corn industries, whose mission is to sell you product, not to provide you and your family with good, quality foods. Big government recommends the engineered stuff over literally everything else. Veggies would make a far healthier foundation.

Despite the Food Pyramid's advice to eat more waffles than spinach, I still believe that the majority of free-thinking, sane-minded individuals see eye to eye on the consumption of produce. The subject of meat is clearly more

The Food Pyramid (or Pyramid of Corruption, as I like to call it).

controversial. I myself believe that we *benefit* from eating muscle: specifically, big-ass T-bone steaks, shrimp cocktail, baby-back ribs. Mankind has been eating meat since we could craft tools and fire. I understand that not everybody loves it like I do, so I speak only for myself as I dissect these sacred pounds of flesh.

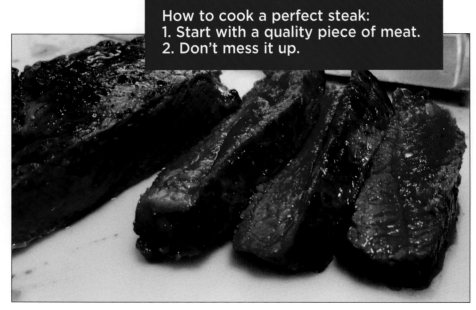

How to cook a perfect steak:
1. Start with a quality piece of meat.
2. Don't mess it up.

You are what you eat. Muscle is made of muscle. While an enormous part of sculpting the shredded six-pack of your dreams means maintaining low body fat, if your abdominal muscles are not built up to a certain degree, there will be nothing to show, despite your leanness. Muscle mass is made of protein. Your abs are made of muscle. Build quality muscle by eating it.

Organ meats are good for you as well. Heart, marrow, tongue and more are on the menu when Danny's in town! In most cultures throughout history, very little of an animal is discarded. The whole beast is used or eaten. (Contemporary America is an exception.) There is richness, nutrition and vitality in animal organs that cannot be found elsewhere. Why do ya' think they call it *liver*? This stuff keeps you alive. Eat organs!

Animal flesh not only tastes delicious, but also satisfies a primal urge to rip meat from bone. Absorb the soul. There's nothing like food with a face! I regularly eat eggs and dairy as well. Yogurt is great, but be mindful of added sugar.

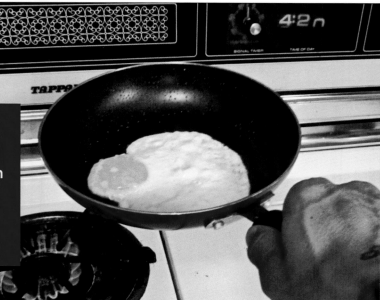

Amazingly there are still people who discard egg yolks—the healthiest part of the egg—because they were misinformed in the 80's. To me this represents over-compartmentalization at its worst. If you choose to eat eggs, then eat eggs. Any questions?

Yes, like grains, the consumption of animal products is every individual's choice. (Never try to convert a vegetarian!) It's also easy to overdo. As much of a carnivore as I am, meat rarely takes up more than a third of my dinner plate. Modern technology has made animal products constantly available to us. In the wild, flesh is much more difficult to earn, as you'd have to kill it, prep it and cook it. Our biology doesn't know that these foods are no longer scarce or time consuming. A large part of abs comes down to being free of gratuitous body weight so restraint is key. Over-eating anything detracts from our mission.

I also eat cheese. I like the good stuff like grass fed Jarlseburg, buffalo mozzarella and local Vermont cheddar. (For the record, the items "cheese food", "cheese product" and "cheez" are not cheese.) When selecting packaged cheese in the supermarket, look at the ingredients. Real cheese usually does not have much more than milk, salt, cheese culture.

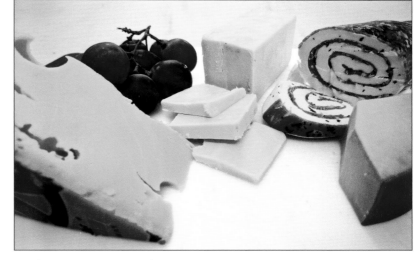

Although there is no denying that countries with obesity rates far lower than the USA (France and Italy for example) consume lots of real cheese, cheese does not agree with everyone.

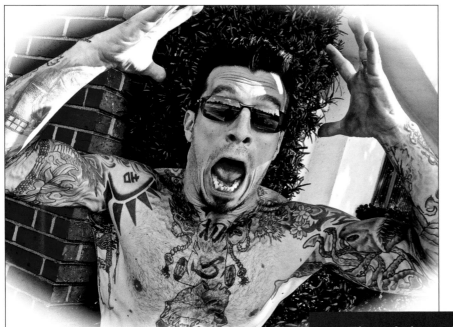

Like many things, the conflicting expert testimony regarding dairy products brings many questions to the table. These questions can be added to the list: Are grains toxic? Is coffee good or bad? Are vegans healthier? Should I eat three squares or six small meals? Do the printed labels "organic" or "free range" really mean anything? What's an anti-oxidant? Does it matter? Aaaarrgghh... the world may never know.

There is lots of conflicting information out there. It can be confusing, even maddening.

Although I think in terms of foods rather than nutrients, it is impossible to discuss animal food products in this century without also mentioning protein. When I was coming up, consuming one and a half to two times the number of grams of protein as your body weight in pounds was recommended for building muscle. (Slightly less is recommended these days.) In other words, if you weighed 180 lbs, you would want anywhere from 270 to 360 grams of protein every day. I vehe-

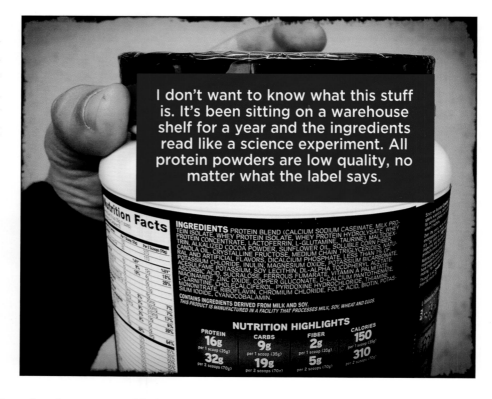

I don't want to know what this stuff is. It's been sitting on a warehouse shelf for a year and the ingredients read like a science experiment. All protein powders are low quality, no matter what the label says.

mently disagree. That is a bunch of crap most likely perpetrated by the supplement industry. If you are not a body-builder, or at least training, eating and dehydrating like one, then protein supplements (like all supplements) are not necessary. That's right. Your body cannot even process such a reckless amount of protein in the first place. You will not get abs from eating this stuff. It's high in calories, and like other supplemental products, low in quality, despite any contrary claims made by paid endorsers, athletes or bogus TV doctors. If you want abs, have a real dinner and skip the protein shake. I'll choose grilled chicken and spinach, with black beans, over a factory-synthesized mixture every single time.

Furthermore, you don't even need *that* much protein in the first place. Protein probably makes up less than a third of my diet. If you want abs, I recommend staying away from all shakes, whether they're ice cream or protein powder. They are both equally detrimental to getting lean. The few times that I deviate from this rule, I choose the ice cream. It's much more worthwhile.

I eat lobster, steak, leafy greens, beats, apples, bananas, peanut butter, chicken, fish, tomatoes, nuts, berries, black beans, garlic, tuna and herbs. Call it what you will: Paleo, Primal, Primitive, Caveman, Low Grain, Mostly Plants, Warrior or whatever: While some of these "name" diets make dubious distinctions from one other (nuts or no nuts?), these brands have more in common than apart. Eating natural, clean foods is a great way to go! Combine this eating style with the right exercise program, and you'll be on your way to rocking a ripped six-pack that's carved out o' wood!

Macronutrients Broken Down

Most nutrients are categorized as carbohydrates, fats or protein. Water is the most important nutrient of all. Time to get technical.

CARBOMANIA

A carbohydrate is an organic compound consisting only of carbon, hydrogen and oxygen. The main sources of carbohydrates are starch and sugars. Sources include starchy vegetables, grains, cereals and legumes. Carbohydrates are often categorized as simple or complex, although I believe this distinction is ambiguous and irrelevant. Either way, most carbohydrates get converted to glucose (sugar) and absorbed into the blood stream, where they can be used as an effective source of energy (or a potential gateway to obesity). Most Americans eat an awful lot of carbohydrates, even more than is usually over-recommended.

THE SKINNY ON FAT

Fat provides buoyancy to the skin, protects the vital organs, and is used as energy. In fact, it's the number one source of stored energy, as evidenced by how much extra fat so many of us are carrying around. Yet unlike carbohydrates, fats are essential. We hear talk of "good" fats and "bad" fats, saturated and unsaturated, mono and poly. Although these distinctions are helpful to some, I've always found them confusing. Lets keep it simple. Fats and oils that exist naturally or with minimal processing (coconut, olive, avocado, peanut, salmon, even butter, bacon and more) are a better choice than the ones made in a lab (corn, soy, soya, canola, anything with the word "hydrogenated").

PROTEIN DREAMS

I don't even think the USDA has a "required" amount of protein. Good; they should adapt that standard for all nutrients. Protein builds and repairs our abs, as well as all muscle and organs in the body, including our hearts and brains. Our bodies digest protein by breaking it down into smaller chemical components called amino acids. There are said to be twenty-two essential amino acids. Animal proteins such as beef, fish, eggs and dairy are considered "complete" because they have all twenty-two. Other protein sources like seeds, black beans and lentils are deemed "incomplete", but with the right combination, this is a non-issue. I've met a lot of muscular vegans in my day.

LET'S GET HYDRATED!

Water removes toxins from the body, improves metabolic rate and digestion, increases energy, helps build muscle, moisturizes the skin and tastes delicious. Water is made of two hydrogen atoms and one oxygen, hence the name H_2O. You and I are made up mostly of water. So is our planet. We can all stand to drink more of it.

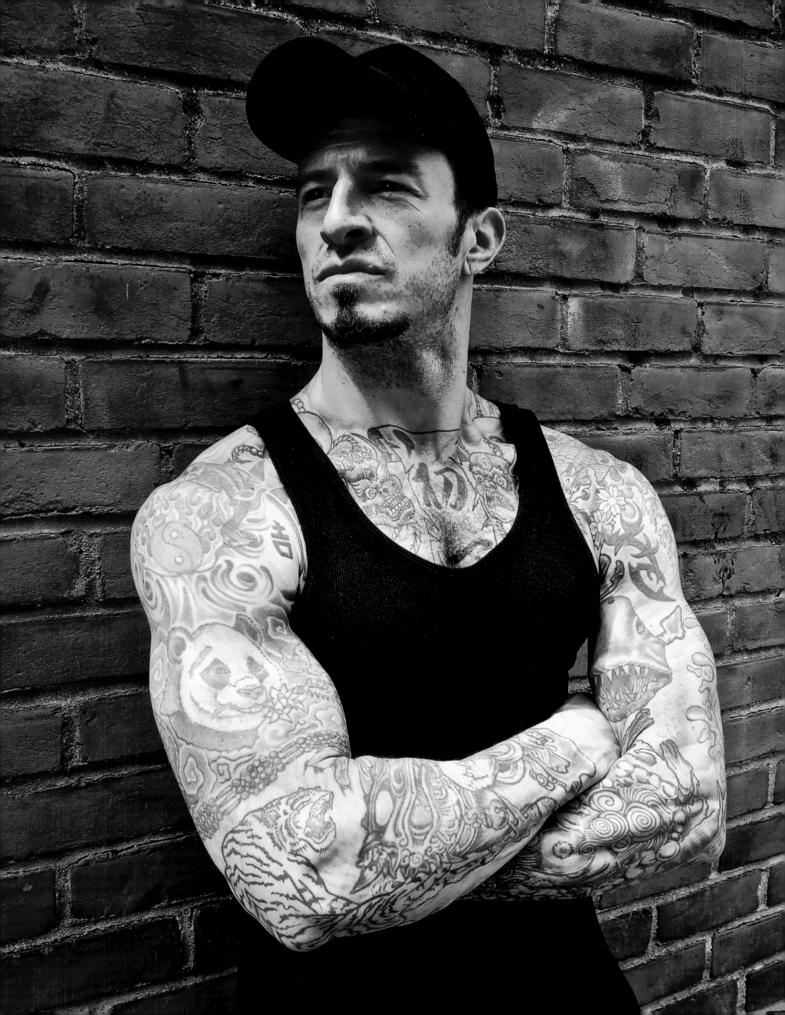

CHAPTER 6

WEIGHING IN ON WEIGHT LOSS

Fact: you cannot own a rock hard set of Diamond-Cut Abs unless you are lean. This means that the ratio of fatty tissue to muscle tissue in your body is low, a state often referred to as "low body fat." For many people, accomplishing this goal requires losing weight. Targeting the belly area with exercise will not reduce the fat. No one wants to believe this but it is true. Fat is reduced throughout the entire body by building muscle, expending more energy and consuming less food. There is no miracle, no secret technique or product.

Furthermore, it is impossible to accurately predict the areas that will lose the fat first. Meaning, we reduce some body fat from the legs, the back, the abs, the neck, etc. It's different for everybody. It can even be different for the same individual, at different times in their life.

We shed body fat only when it is metabolized for fuel. A constantly full stomach will prevent this from happening. Moving, exercising and other types of physical exertion cause us to metabolize food for energy. When we are depleted of energy sources including stored glycogen, we delve into body fat.

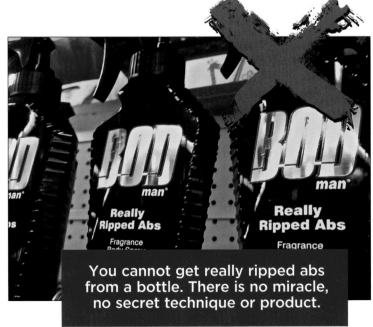

You cannot get really ripped abs from a bottle. There is no miracle, no secret technique or product.

Though it's completely possible to get impeccable abs without ever measuring your body fat (I haven't measured mine in years), some people find the numbers helpful. If this pertains to you, then please understand that most available methods of measuring your body fat percentage are mere estimates at best. That said, if you are training intensely and consistently, then the difference between Diamond-Cut Abs and what my friends and I used to call "four-cubes-and-a-gut" comes down to having an *extremely* low body fat (single digit for the men, teens or less for the women), as opposed to simply having a low one (under 15% for men, under 25% for women). Like it or not, this usually comes down to food intake. You cannot train your way out of bad eating habits.

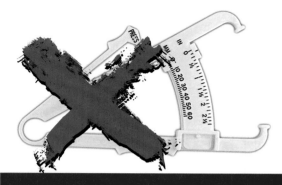

Body fat testers like these calipers provide a rough estimate at best. It's nearly impossible to get a completely accurate reading. Let's not get hung up on numbers, man.

It is important to note that the "fat content" of a food or food product has no bearing on if it will be converted to body fat. Everything that is not used for fuel gets stored as fat. (That's one more reason to avoid those 700-calorie post-workout shakes in favor of water if you want abs.)

The word "calorie" refers to a kilocalorie (Kcal). It is a measurement of heat-- how much energy is needed to "burn off" a carrot or a donut or two ice cream bars. If I use 3,000 calories in a day due to energy expenditure, training, muscle mass and metabolism, and I only consume 2,000, I will lose weight. (This formula is referred to as Calories in/Calories Out, or being in a "caloric deficit".) Do the math; it works. That's also part of why the low grain thing works. Many Americans eat two dinner rolls before their appetizer, then a meal, complete with French fried potatoes, rice and a glass of Coca-Cola. Cutting the sugar and grains leaves *plenty* of room for greens, hence cutting the overall caloric intake dramatically. (Substituting veggies for rolls and water for Coke also brings a great deal more nutrients to the table... again, common sense!)

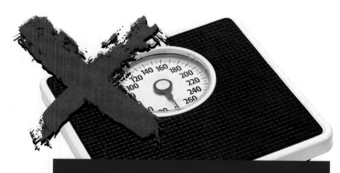

Blow up your scale. I haven't weighed myself in years and would not care if the scale read 125 or 225 lbs. However, if you feel that you absolutely must weigh yourself, I implore you to do so once a week or less. Keep the scale in the closet and out of sight. Daily weigh-ins are part of the recipe for disaster.

That's one of the reasons why thinking in terms of foods rather than calories is extremely effective for weight loss, as it is for overall health. For me, and almost everyone I know with amazing abs, it makes more sense than counting calories, and requires neither a chart nor calculator. Yes, some folks prefer to visualize numbers, but I have not observed that to be a formula for long term success; it's no way to live.

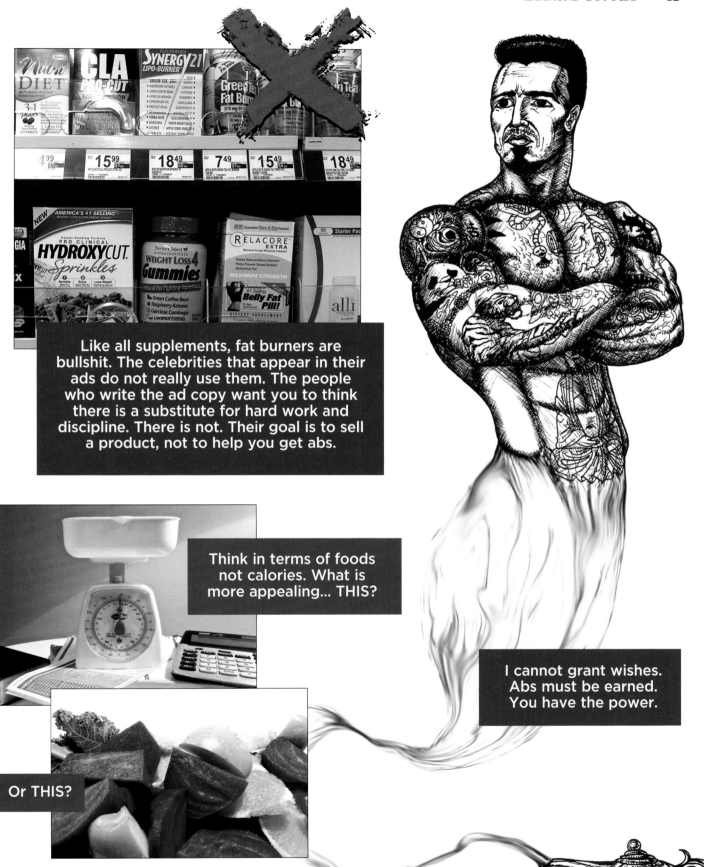

Like all supplements, fat burners are bullshit. The celebrities that appear in their ads do not really use them. The people who write the ad copy want you to think there is a substitute for hard work and discipline. There is not. Their goal is to sell a product, not to help you get abs.

Think in terms of foods not calories. What is more appealing... THIS?

I cannot grant wishes. Abs must be earned. You have the power.

Or THIS?

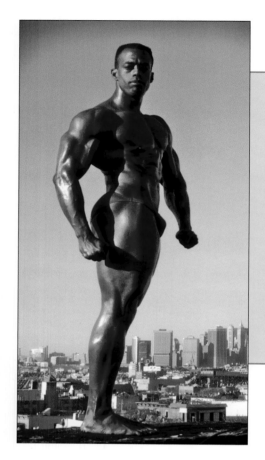

Is This Man Obese?

Shockingly, according to Body Mass Index (BMI), he is. I believe BMI should be called B.S.MI because it's bullshit. This flawed and antiquated system is used in many institutions that people trust, including the World Health Organization, most commercial training facilities and even our own public schools. B.S.MI is calculated solely from numeric measurements of weight and height. It does not take any other factors (like body composition, lifestyle or in this case, simple observation) into account. Based on B.S.MI, a body-builder would be considered obese. Once again, I advise paying less attention to numbers and more attention to our senses.

When it comes to getting ripped, sometimes you have to be hungry. Assuming that I have an *average* daily intake of about 3,000 calories, it's still very seldom that I get exactly 3,000 in any single day. For example, Monday I may have numerous personal training clients and be out and about from 6am-8pm, commuting by bicycle. Perhaps I only have coffee, water, bananas and nuts on this day, consuming barely 1,000 calories. That's good. It keeps me lean. On the other hand, I have days like Thanksgiving where my caloric intake is six times that, and far exceeds my energy expenditure. Basically what I'm saying, is, *Don't be afraid to be hungry.* It's okay. So many people have no problem being stuffed, but they feel like they're jeopardizing their health if they're hungry for any duration of time. Let yourself get hungry if you're gonna let yourself get full. Find the balance. If you having pig-out days once or twice a week, be prepared to counter them with one or two fruit-n-veggie days too. Sometimes it's better to consider your food intake over several days, rather than making daily restrictions. Not every day is exactly the same, nor should they be. That's what makes life beautiful.

The reality of obtaining ripped abs sometimes means sacrifice. Sacrifices can make you strong, not just in a physical sense. Giving into every whim is neither mentally nor spiritually healthy.

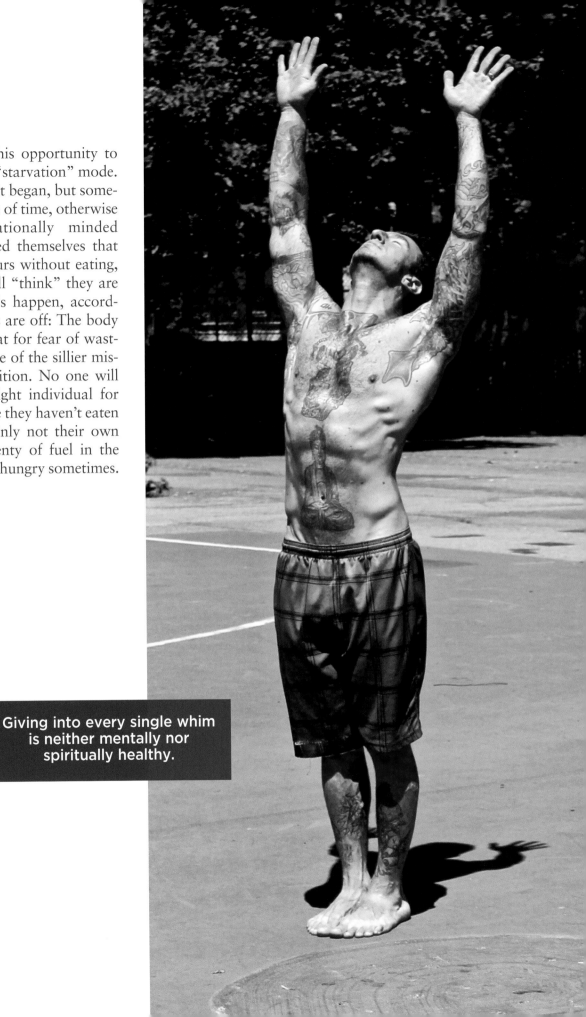

I'd like to take this opportunity to discuss the myth of "starvation" mode. I do not know how it began, but somehow, over the course of time, otherwise intelligent and rationally minded grown-ups convinced themselves that if they go a few hours without eating, that their bodies will "think" they are starving. Should this happen, according to myth, all bets are off: The body will hold on to its fat for fear of wasting away. This is one of the sillier misconceptions in nutrition. No one will mistake an overweight individual for starving just because they haven't eaten since brunch, certainly not their own body! They got plenty of fuel in the tank. It's okay to be hungry sometimes.

Giving into every single whim is neither mentally nor spiritually healthy.

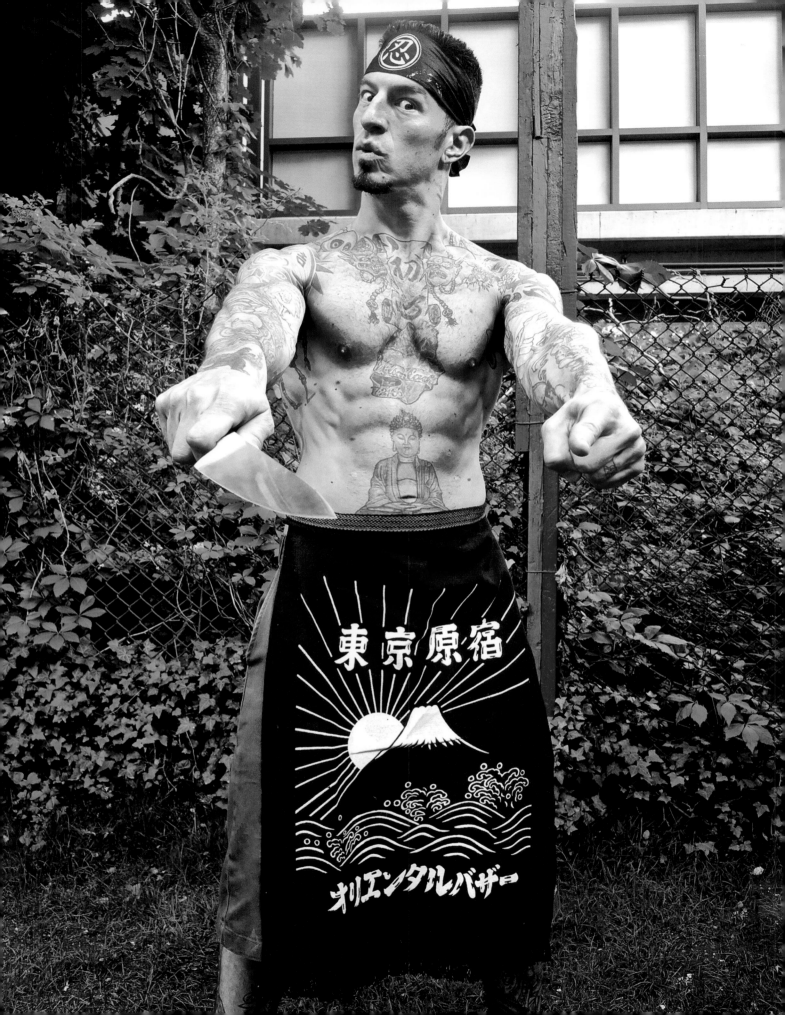

CHAPTER 7

WHAT I EAT

People always ask me what I eat. They want specifics. Here are some answers: Apples, onions, garlic, olive oil, broccoli, nuts, spinach, fish, crustaceans, herbs, beef, butter, peppers, peanut butter, chickpeas, chicken (skin on), carrots, eggs, bacon, and a whole lot more. I eat Brussels sprouts, avocados, cheese, pork chops and corn on the cob. There are even times when I eat pizza or bake cookies, just not most of the time. The notion that people with a six-pack live in a state of perpetual deprivation is a bunch of hooey. The fittest people I know eat whole, delicious, flavorful foods pretty much whenever they want. To paraphrase Mark Sisson in The Primal Blueprint, I eat a diet consisting of mostly plants and animals. Notice I said "mostly". That's because if you eat well most of the time, there are no foods that you'll always have to avoid forever. Just keep yourself in check.

I love to prepare food.

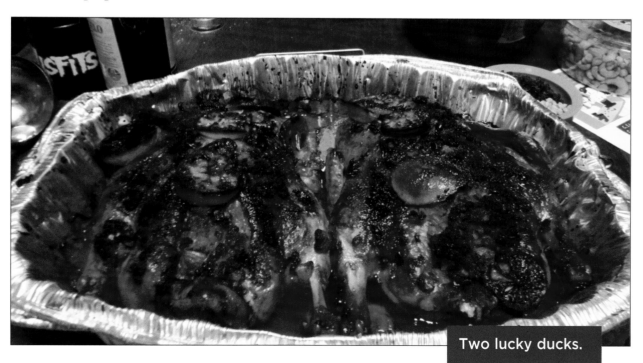

Two lucky ducks.

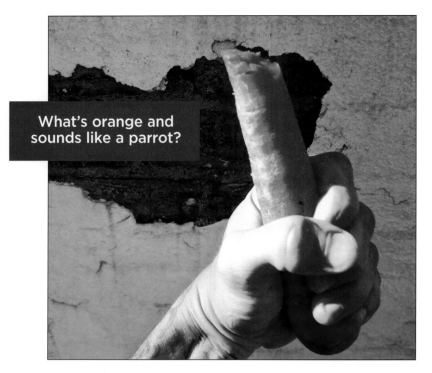

What's orange and sounds like a parrot?

I like cooking my meat on the bone. I use as few ingredients as necessary. I prefer produce to be as close to the source as possible and never overdone. I enjoy eating with people I care about.

Food preparation really is all about care. It involves being in the present moment. If I'm peeling garlic, every little clove gets my love and undivided attention. My eyes and hands do not wander. When I grill a steak, I'm right there with it. I never phone it in. I approach my recipes like my workouts. I keep them in the present. Taste the food. Touch it. Go with the flow. Cook with flavors and spices that make you feel alive.

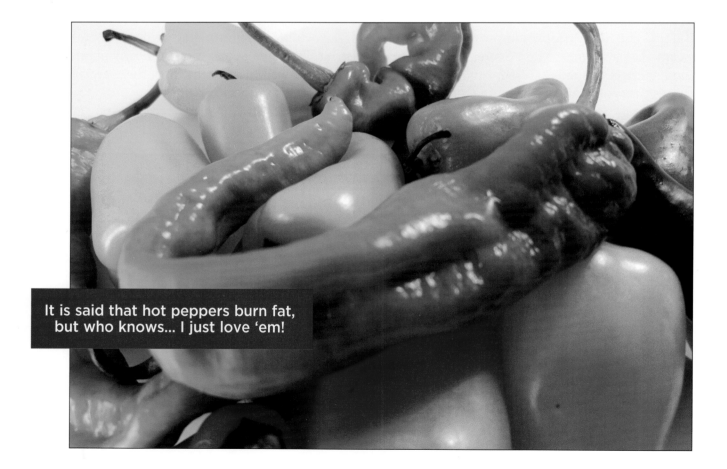

It is said that hot peppers burn fat, but who knows... I just love 'em!

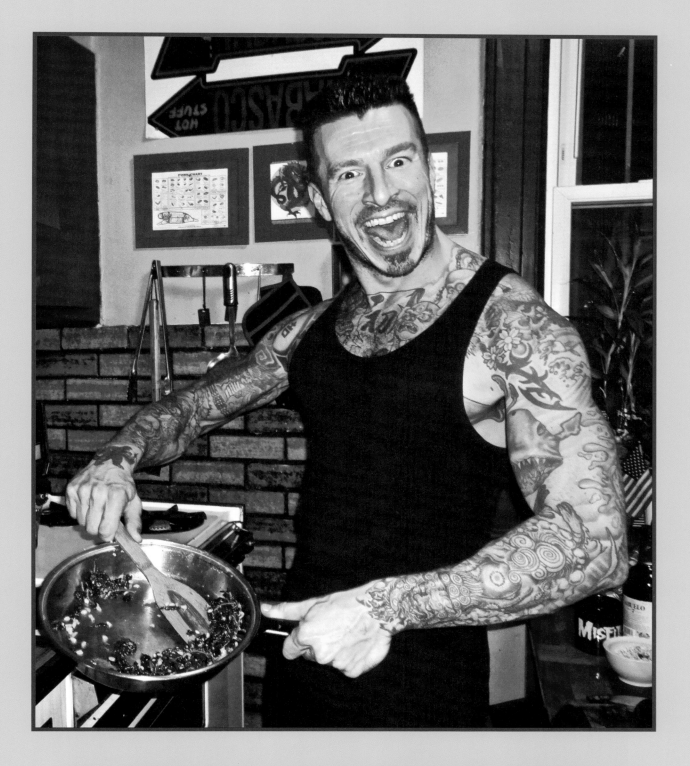

"Approach love and cooking with reckless abandon."
–Dalai Lama

Don't be afraid to improvise when you cook. Suit recipes to taste. Enjoy seasonal ingredients. I believe that cooking should be like making love. YES, although you know what generally works, strictly adhering to a plan just ain't as good as being in the present moment. Love your food!

3-Day Sample Food Log

Here is a look at what I might consume over the course of three days:

DAY 1

Pre-Breakfast: Coffee, Milk
Breakfast: Apples, oranges, plums
Lunch: Big chef salad—veggies and meat
Dinner: Steak, broccoli, corn salsa, wine
Snack: Bananas and peanut butter
Note: Water consumed all day

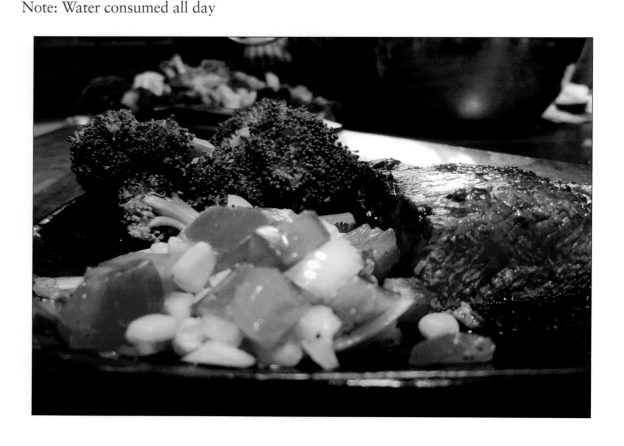

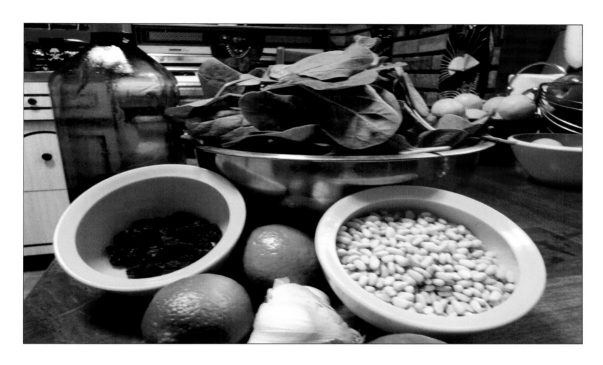

DAY 2

Pre-Breakfast: Coffee, Milk
Breakfast: Fresh Juice (See Chapter 8 for examples.)
Snack: Peapods
Lunch: Cheeseburger and salad
Dinner: Spinach olive oil, pine nuts, raisins
Snack: Almonds and blueberries
Note: Fruit and water consumed all day

DAY 3

Pre-Breakfast: Coffee, Milk
Breakfast: Bacon, eggs, cheese, juice
Lunch: Salmon sashimi, edamame, seaweed, avocado
Dinner: Lamb chops and greens
Snack: Carrots, celery, peppers, hummus, cashews
Note: Fruit and water consumed all day

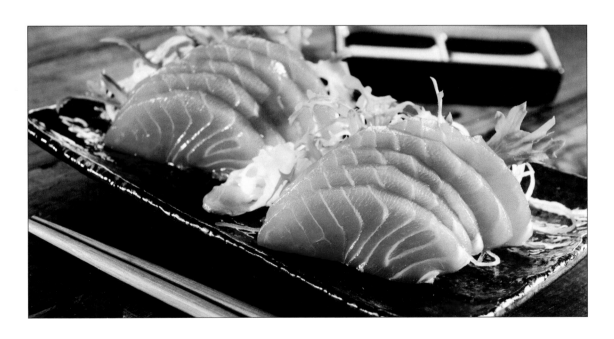

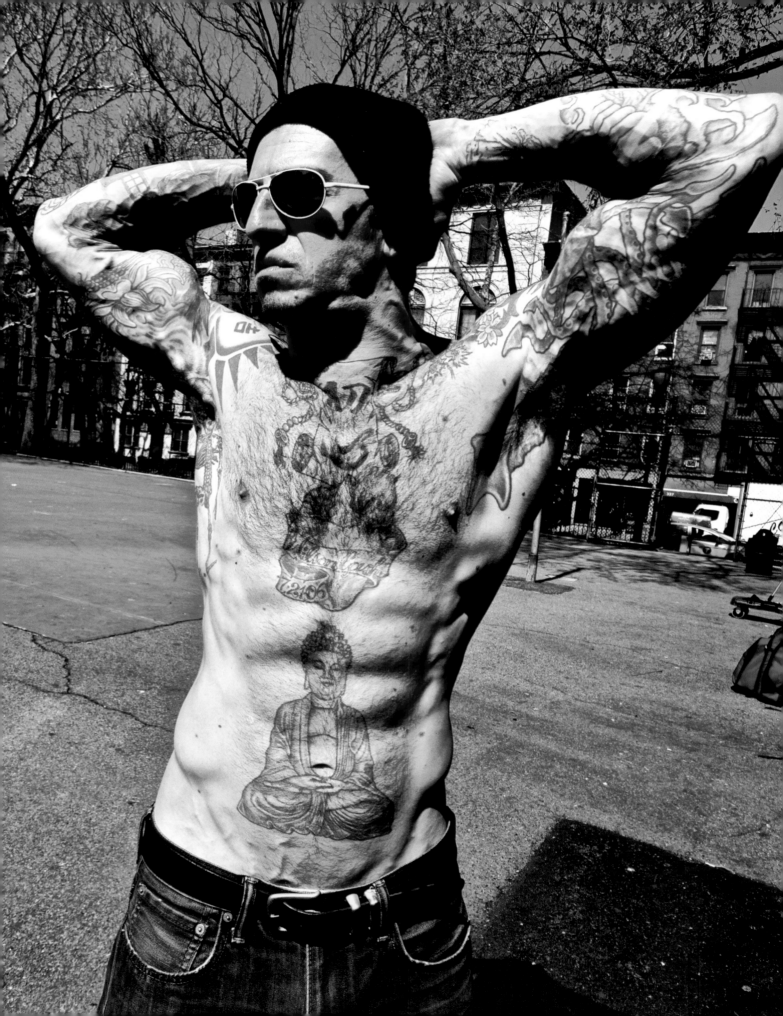

CHAPTER 8

THE FAST AND THE CURIOUS

When I was in seventh grade, during a lecture about digestion, my science teacher Mr. Yorx said "After about twelve hours on an empty stomach, your body starts to digest stored fat". While I doubted that this statement was 100% true to the letter, the premise made sense to me. It still does.

In recent years, fasting has been getting a lot of attention. Several internet fasts have gone viral and numerous brands of cleanses have entered the marketplace. As the benefits of fasting garner more acknowledgement than ever before, it's natural for some of us to be a little curious.

You see, the digestive system never gets much of a break. Seriously, many folks rarely go even twelve hours without eating... they're constantly "backed up". In fact, the average American has about eight pounds of shit in their digestive tract at all times. That's part of the reason why the words "fast" and "cleanse" are sometimes used interchangeably.

As far as your abs are concerned, although you will get a bit leaner after almost any fast, this short term reduction in body fat shouldn't be the primary motivation. To me, the fact that fasting places an individual at a great starting point toward eating mindfully and healthfully *moving forward after the fast* is far more important. It's like hitting a "RESET" button on your appetite and eating habits. At the completion of a fast, not only is your colon empty, but your whole way of thinking about food has been altered, at least temporarily.

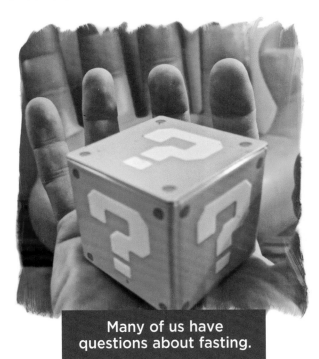

Many of us have questions about fasting.

The concept of intermittent fasting is not new at all. Ritual fasting has existed in many cultures throughout mankind's history. Heck, we all fast every single night. That's why the first meal of the day is called "break fast".

Technically, Merriam-Webster's Dictionary defines "fast" as

1. *To abstain from food.*
2. *To eat sparingly or abstain from some foods.*

So, fasting means that one abstain fully (or in part) from some (or all) foods (and/or drinks). There is a lot of room for interpretation here. Technically, going grain free, dairy free, vegan and more, could all be considered forms of fasts. (I personally fancy them to be "eating styles" but what's in a name?) That said, there are still many types of fasts. Here are some examples. With the exception of the Absolute Fast, (which I do not generally recommend), be sure to consume plenty of water when embarking on any of them.

BEGINNERS' CLEANSE

If you've never had any dietary restrictions at all, then this is where you start. Ease in by eliminating sugar, added salt, alcohol and caffeine, as well as all packaged and processed foods from the time you wake up until the time you go to bed. If it feels good, try to hold out for two or three days and re-assess. Many of us sustain this or a similar eating style for life.

That's how it begins.

If this goes well, then next time you attempt the Beginners' Cleanse, take out a little bit more. Try eliminating all grains (breads, cereals and pasta for example) for anywhere from one to three days.

By your third or fourth attempt, eliminate all meat, including fish and dairy. The goal is to get to the point where you

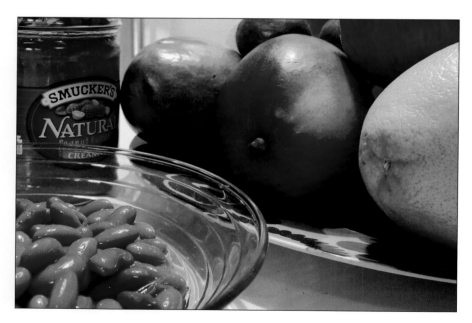

can eat mostly fruits and vegetables, nuts, seeds, legumes for two or three days. I don't recommend any beverages other than water, homemade vegetable broth and herbal tea. Naturally, now would be a great time to get acquainted with freshly made juices.

Notice that I did not say "freshly squeezed juices". While I highly recommend eating whole fruits, some of them (citrus for example) need their natural pulp to help regulate the absorption of sugar. Because we want to avoid sugar, I recommend *juicing* fruits and vegetables (such as carrots, spinach, apples, beets, herbs), rather than *squeezing* them.

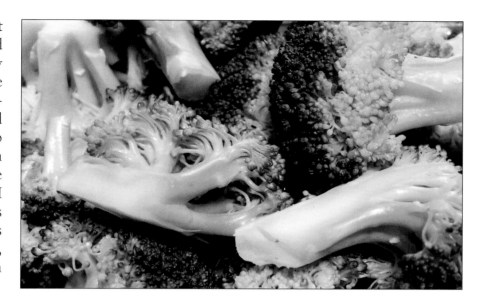

For those used to eating all foods in abundance, then just these changes will probably be difficult. Others will find it more appropriate to start with the Fruit N Veggie Cleanse.

FRUIT N VEGGIE CLEANSE

At the time of this writing, I have fasted on and off to varying degrees for the past fifteen years. I still do a Fruit N Veggie Cleanse somewhat frequently, typically for one to three days. One could do a Fruit N Veggie Cleanse indefinitely, just not me.

Like the Beginner's Cleanse, the law of the Fruit N Veggie Cleanse is not carved in stone. You can go strict Fruit N Veggie, consuming nothing but fruits, vegetables, water, juice and tea. Or you can add nuts, nut butters, beans, seeds and legumes. I recommend plenty of vegetable based fats like olive oil and

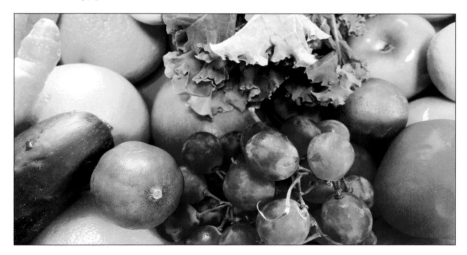

avocados. When doing a Fruit N Veggie Cleanse, try to get as many different colors and flavors of succulent fruits and vegetables as possible.

If you're used to eating a lot of starch, you will be hungry frequently, so be prepared for an exercise in restraint. Have as much produce on hand as possible and lay it out so it looks beautiful. Take a bag of carrots, green beans or apples with you when you leave the house. This foresight will help alleviate temptation.

Don't be surprised if you sweat and stink a bit after the first few days. That's good. It means the bad stuff is leaving the body.

JUICE FAST

Now we're talking.

My definition of a Juice Fast is a bit stricter than my definitions of previous cleanses. It includes freshly made juices, water, vegetable broth and herbal tea. Of course, if you're starving and *REALLY* need a banana, then have one—it doesn't mean you failed. But please understand, a Juice Fast requires a level of willpower that many folks have never tapped into before in their lives.

The occasional juice fast does wonders. As you flush your body (and soul!) with highly concentrated vitamins, minerals and enzymes, you also give your digestive system some much needed down time. Several years ago, I did four Juice Fasts, one at the change of each season. It was awesome.

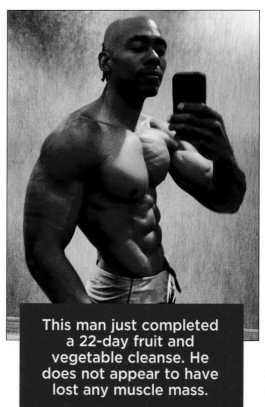

This man just completed a 22-day fruit and vegetable cleanse. He does not appear to have lost any muscle mass.

I don't follow a specific menu program when juice fasting. I simply try to get as many extraordinary colors and flavors as possible. Be leery of overly restrictive juice fasts. I personally shy away from anything that says to consume *"nothing but"* their particular brand of juices or jacked-up cayenne pepper lemonade. Further, there is no reason to split hairs over what time of day and how much of each juice is consumed. A Juice Fast in itself is restrictive enough! I prefer having as many juices as I want, whenever I choose. A juice fast is not the same as a crash diet, nor should it be.

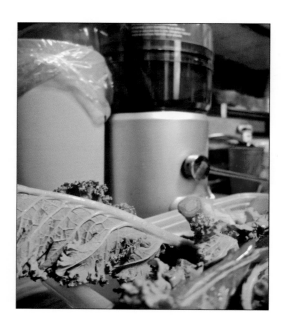

It may behoove you to do a Fruit N Veggie Cleanse before *and* after a Juice Fast to help ease you in and out. A nice seven-day plan is a two day Fruit N Veggie "Pre-Fast", followed by a three day Juice Fast, concluding with another Fruit N Veggie "Post-Fast". You won't look at food again the same way for a long time.

It is important to note, as opponents of fasting often do, that in spite of its numerous benefits, not much fiber is consumed during a juice fast, making it potentially difficult for the body to rid itself of built-up toxins after the first few days. Some proponents of fasting swear by the colonic or enema, both of which are obviously very personal choices. Although there is no doubt that either will solve the waste management issue, neither is necessarily called for. Every individual and every fast is different.

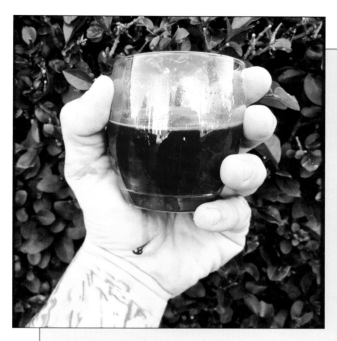

Danny's Favorite Juices

My family and I juice almost everyday, having nothing to do with fasting. We buy the produce, lay it out and look at the colors. We touch the food, chop it up and juice it. This ritual is both calming and exciting at the same time.

These are some of my favorite recipes. They are delicious and balance each other nicely. Please mix 'em up, change 'em around, add or take away. If you want to put apples in your Leafy Green Juice, then do it! Don't forget, you don't need to be on a cleanse to celebrate the goodness of fresh juice anytime!

1. **Leafy Green Juice**
   Spinach, Kale, Lettuce, Cucumber, Jalapeno, twist of Lemon.

2. **Bloody Mary Juice**
   Tomato, Garlic, Cilantro, Celery, Horseradish, add Black Pepper to taste.

3. **The Classic**
   Carrot, Apple, Ginger.

4. **The Cleanser**
   Beet, Spinach, Apple, Red Pepper, twist of Grapefruit.

TRUE FAST

The True Fast is an extreme exercise in discipline and is absolutely not for everybody. Nothing is consumed in a True Fast except water. For that reason, it is often referred to as a "Water Fast".

Be prepared for a serious mental trip with this fast. Your mind will visit places you have never been and your perception of hunger and appetite will be tested. Whereas all previous fasts allow some sort of consumption of organic matter, the True Fast does not.

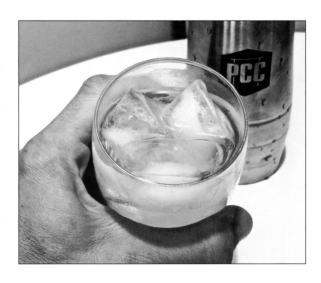

A high level of mental commitment is involved here; you must simply get used to the feeling of constantly being hungry. Accept.

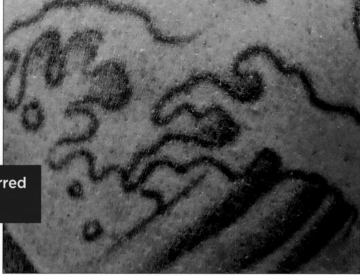

A True Fast is also referred to as a Water Fast.

ABSOLUTE FAST

Technically speaking, an Absolute Fast forbids the consumption of all food and water for at least 24 hours. It is the only fast on this list with which I do not have extensive personal experience. Body builders, fashion models and athletes who compete in weight classes sometimes employ Absolute Fasts as a dehydration technique. Someone on a hunger strike also chooses to do an Absolute Fast.

The human body can go days, even weeks without solid food but it is not healthy to go extended periods of time without water.

Be Steadfast To Your Fast

All of these fasts can be a physical and emotional roller coaster. Here are a few tips for safe and successful fasting:

1. The very beginning can be tough. You may feel light headed or cranky the first day. If possible, try to plan your fast when your schedule is open, especially if it's your first one. Don't physically exert too much until you feel it out.

2. Naturally some moments will be easier than others. Be prepared. You may find yourself experiencing hunger, anger, euphoria or despair at different times. Allow those feelings to exist and to pass. Fasting is a physical and psychological test, like a road trip (or acid trip).

3. When your fast is completed, ease back into the food. For the days or weeks following your fast, you're likely to experience a new appreciation for the simplicity and value of every bite you eat. You'll be amazed at how incredible a single grape can taste, and wonder how you could ever have eaten a heaping mound of chili cheese nachos in your life.

4. Have some fun with it. Completion is its own reward. Drink plenty of water and see what happens. Good luck!

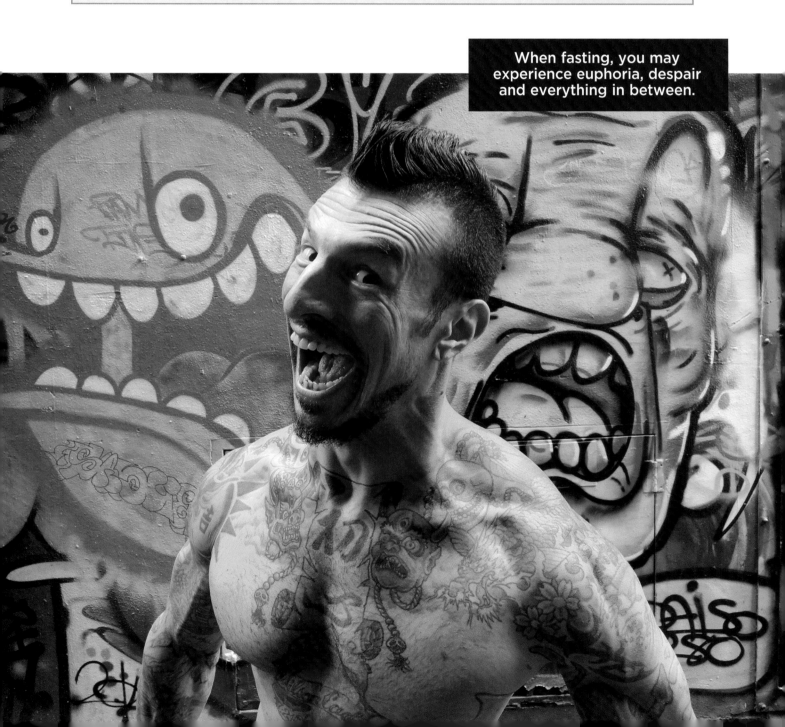

When fasting, you may experience euphoria, despair and everything in between.

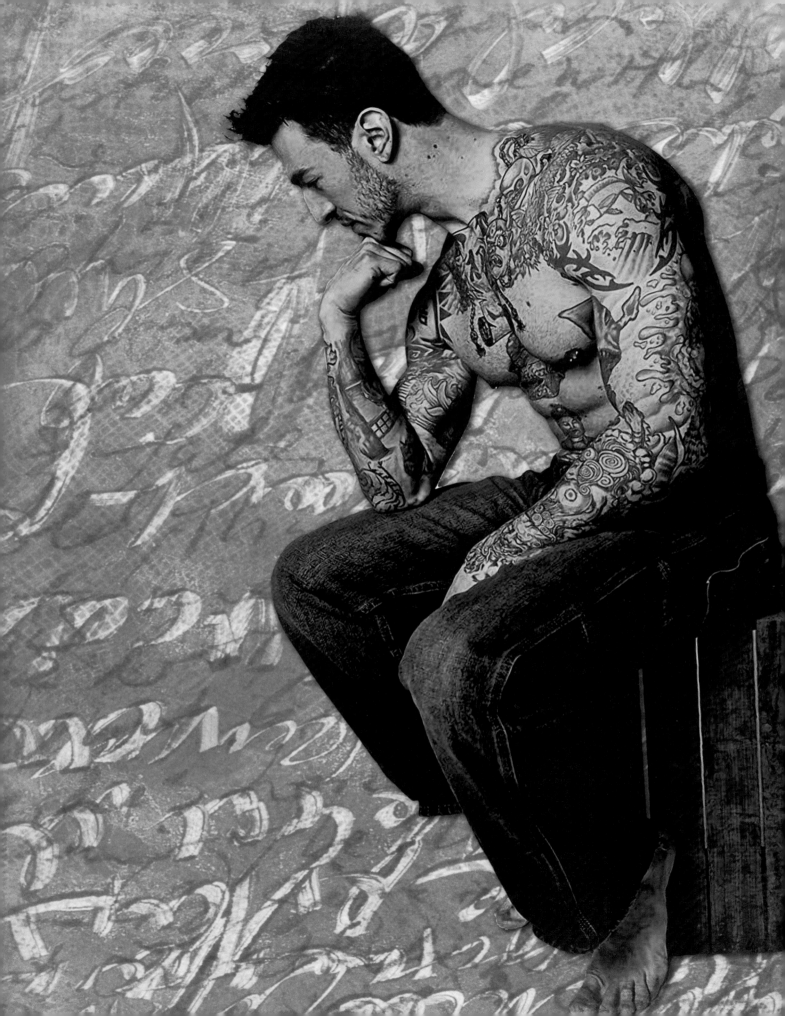

CHAPTER 9

MORE FOOD FOR THOUGHT

We are here to talk about abs, not saving the world. Still, I feel it would be irresponsible to discuss healthy eating in any capacity, without at least mentioning the subject of genetically and chemically modified foods. We consume these foods in the United States of America more than ever. In fact, some foods are nearly impossible to find in their true form. What we call the Western Diet, which is spreading all over the world, is more of an experiment in science and economics than an actual menu.

First things first, I wholeheartedly acknowledge the numerous positives effects of food science and industry, such as stronger crops, greater food distribution and more cost efficient methods. Farming itself is a form of science, so, trust me, no one opposes food science in an absolute sense. But it seems to have run amuck over the past few decades. This is a usual pattern: Something starts out as with noble intentions (Make produce with a greater survival rate or help diminish world hunger), but becomes corrupted over time. As the corporate model grows, the corruption often follows.

You see, food is big business, and the few *major* manufacturers of food in the USA have one, and only one, priority: To make as many dollars as possible. Build a bigger chicken, sell more meat. The chickens we eat are the animal equivalent of a two hundred pound six-year-old child with busted, stunted limbs on an arsenic-laced diet.

The commercial apples we eat are bloated and flaccid, lacking in fiber and overall "apple-y" goodness, compared to the ones grown by smaller farms. They're larger, yet lower in vitality and nutrition. Most of the food consumed in America is manufactured with methods and ingredients that do not keep our best interest in mind. This runs the gamut from harmful chemicals in our produce, to freakish DNA, to unnecessary suffering. Many of the chemicals we don't even test for in our food are banned in hundreds of countries. Additives ranging from coloring agents to arsenic are allowed in the U.S.A, not to mention others not even qualified by the FDA to be identified as ingredients. We do not have the right to know what we're eating in the "Land of the Free".

Many countries don't make the distinction of "organic" produce, "grass fed" beef or "no added hormones" chicken. Why? Because in most of Europe and many other parts of the world, it's *all* organic! How about that?

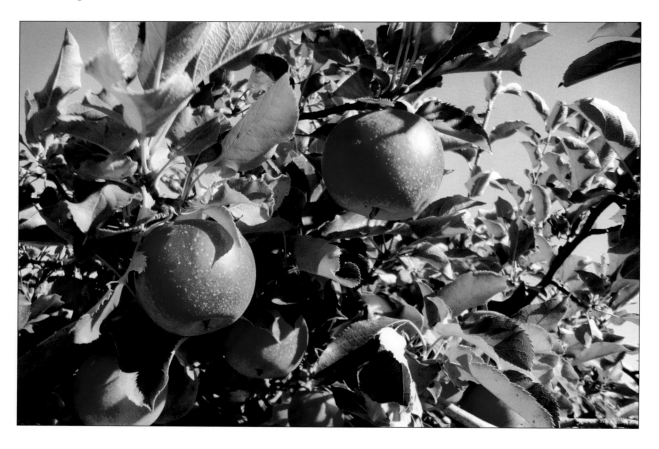

Children Of The Corn

It is alarming how much corn and corn-derived product Americans consume. It is everywhere, whether in the form of corn syrup (which is added to almost everything) or corn fed beef. I'm not talking about sweet, edible yellow corn either, which is delicious any time. I am referring to tough starchy corns concocted and engineered strictly for business purposes—stuff you couldn't eat until it's been chemically rendered and processed. A good rule of thumb is, don't eat the corn if you can't see the corn.

Don't eat the corn if you can't see the corn.

We don't know the long-term effects of the Western Diet, in part because the science and manufacturing of food changes so fast. Even McDonald's wasn't as bad for you twenty-five years ago as it is now. But contrary to what the powers that be will tell you, this is not the only way to eat. Many toxic foods can be avoided. It takes effort, but like all things workout-related, that's a good thing! Shop locally, befriend a farmer and investigate. It may indeed be impossible to eliminate every single questionable element from your diet, but awareness is a great start. Consider this challenge to be an opportunity to learn more about the most important health related decision you can make—what you choose to put in your body.

Beyond the typically low quality, one of the most harmful effects of food technology is simply that we're eating way too much, too often. So much food (much of it questionable) is constantly available at our collective fingertips. Fast food, processed cake treats and soda pop are over-abundant all the time. Even in a health conscious city like New York, where I've resided all my life, there is cheap, processed crap literally around every corner.

Yet, no matter how tough the times (or the government) make it, it is possible to eat well here in the States. We just gotta try a little harder these days.

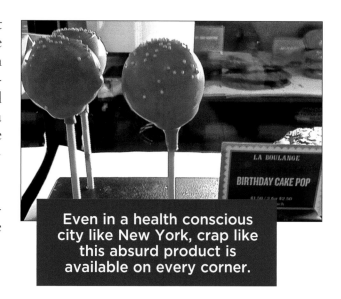

Even in a health conscious city like New York, crap like this absurd product is available on every corner.

Happy Hands

Food has a soul and I like eating it when it's made with love and care. The chef's energy is in the food. Someone who enjoys preparing a meal uses happy hands. A pissed-off fast food worker does not. I avoid angry hands.

To take it another step, food is generally better when made by a human in a kitchen, not by a corporation in a factory. Love is the secret ingredient.

I have love for every single clove of garlic I slice and each guest at my table. You can taste the difference.

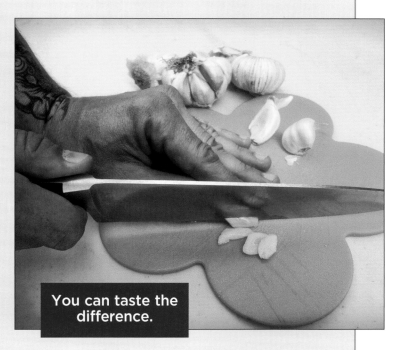

You can taste the difference.

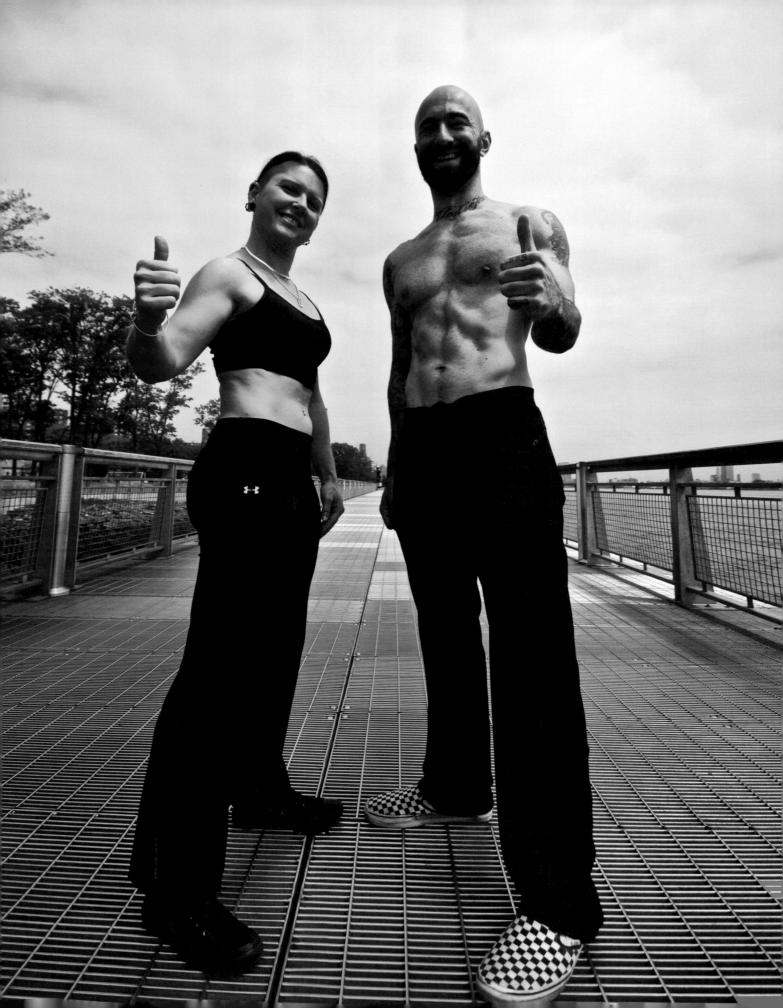

CHAPTER 10

TOP TEN TIPS
for
TIP TOP ABS

There are many dietary principles and practices that contribute to carving out Diamond-Cut Abs. Some of them are more obvious, others sublime. The ones listed here have been proven time and time again to work. Here are my personal top ten tips.

1. Abs are made in the kitchen not the gym.

It's a cliché because it's true. You cannot train your way out of a poor diet. Keep good foods on hand and you're more likely to make sound choices. Cook as many meals as possible; it's the best way to know what you're actually eating. Since being lean is a prerequisite to getting ripped abs, you will have to show some restraint at times. As a general rule, whether it pertains to snacking or the dinner table, we could all probably stand to eat more veggies, less everything else.

2. Eat an orange. Skip the juice.

Fruit gives you abs but squeezed fruit juice can actually prevent it. Fruit juice has all the sugar but none of the fiber. Eat lots of fruit and drink lots of water. Obviously, avoid soda, sugary iced tea beverages and sports drinks too.

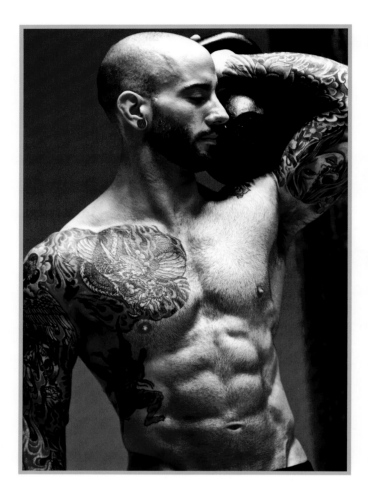

3. Eat less sugar.

Here's a simple one. Stay away from stuff made of sugar—use common sense. Remember organic cane sugar, high fructose corn syrup, honey and agave nectar are all sugar. Your abs don't know the difference. Don't add sugar (or sugar substitutes) to coffee, tea or anything else either. Trust me, your taste buds will adjust in a few days.

4. If you must eat packaged foods, look at ingredients.

A great way to avoid processed, synthetic foods is to stay away from anything with a long list of ingredients that you could not identify in nature, like soy lecithin or anything with the word "syrup". A good rule of thumb is to avoid ingredients that have more than four syllables if you don't know what they are.

5. Drink more water, less everything else.

The importance of drinking water cannot be overstated, particularly as it relates to your abs. Among other things, water removes the byproducts of fat and improves metabolic rate and digestion. This helps you get leaner. Water also moisturizes, increasing your skin's suppleness, thereby enhancing your abs's appearance. It removes toxins and reduces aches and pains, helping you to train harder and more consistently. Water is a friend of abs. (This does not include flavored water, vitamin water or the like. Carbonated is fine.)

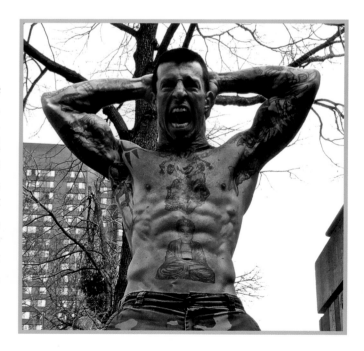

6. "Low-fat" foods do not mean low-fat you.

Be dubious of any food that makes a blatant health claim like "low-fat", "low-sugar", "gluten free" or "all natural". Although theoretically these sentiments appear desirable, generally food products that advertise themselves as such compensate by adding chemicals and artificial ingredients to what is usually already an extremely low quality product. I make it a practice to steer clear of almost any item that make any health claims at all. When a phrase like "sugar free" is the best a food conglomerate's legal team can do to convince you that their products will not kill you, then perhaps it's best to avoid the product in the first place.

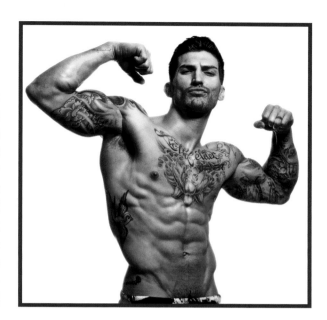

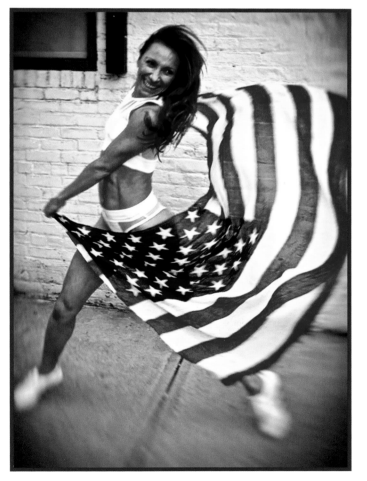

7. Have your condiments on the side.

Many condiments are candy. Much of the ketchup, BBQ sauce, mayonnaise and marinades on your grocer's shelves are nothing more than gratuitous chemicals and calories. This is not to say they must be avoided altogether, but rather, consumed with mindfulness. Even salad dressing is tricky. Unless you made it yourself, dipping your salad in dressing is a better practice than slathering it all over. Better yet, skip the dressing and opt for some vinegar and olive oil. Crack some black pepper. Go crazy.

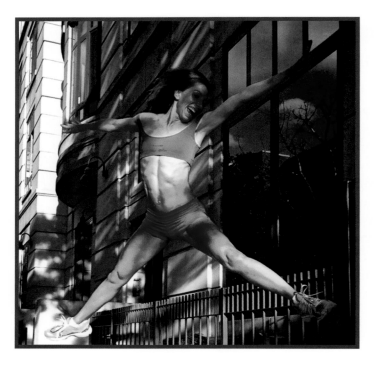

8. Supplements are bullshit.

I do not use or endorse any supplements whatsoever. I am referring to all protein powders, vitamins, extracts, fat burners, etc. That's right, all of them, even "natural" ones. Save your money. They don't work. Everything is better when it comes from the source and all supplements are low quality, no matter what the ad copy says. They have no place in our diet.

9. Eating for weight loss is not the same as eating for maintenance.

When the goal is to drop body fat or get lighter, essentially making less you, you will have to eat with more restrictions than when you are trying to maintain the same weight and not reduce your body mass. That's just the way it is. Mostly, this simply comes down to eating less when you are trying to lose weight. No tricks.

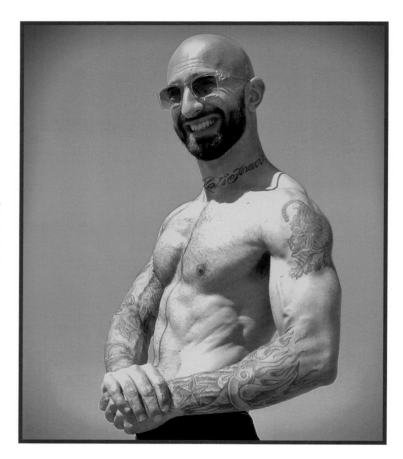

10. You can eat like a fat guy but you can't eat like two fat guys.

There are no foods that we must literally avoid 100% of the time. You can enjoy an occasional bacon cheeseburger and still maintain a set of Diamond-Cut Abs. I do. However, that succulent burger is where it ends. With it, I generally get a salad, not fries. I drink water, not soda. I eat like one fat guy, not two.

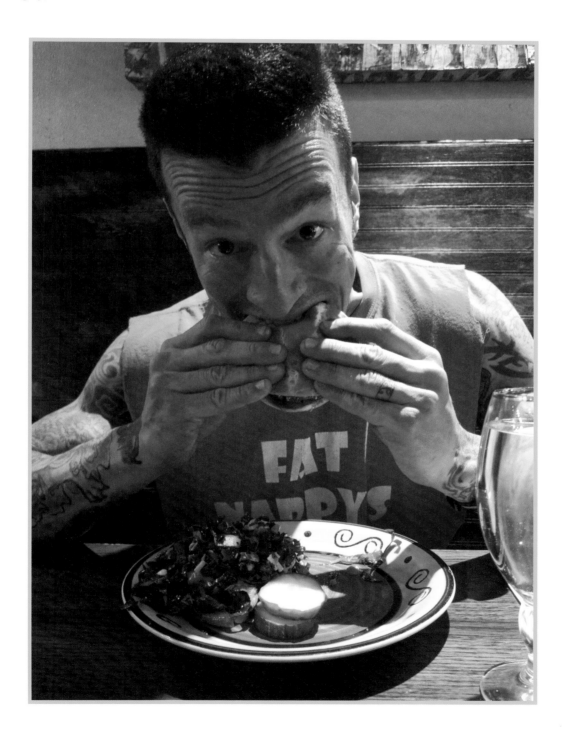

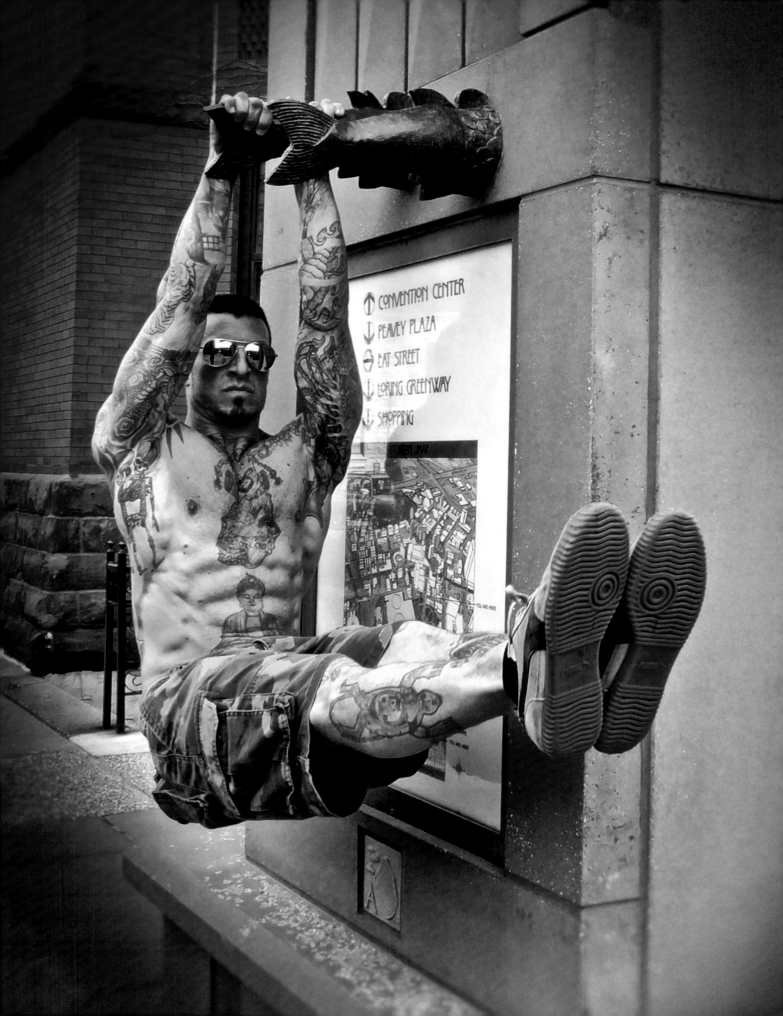

PART III

TRAINING YOUR ABS

"Honesty Is My Only Excuse."
–Metallica

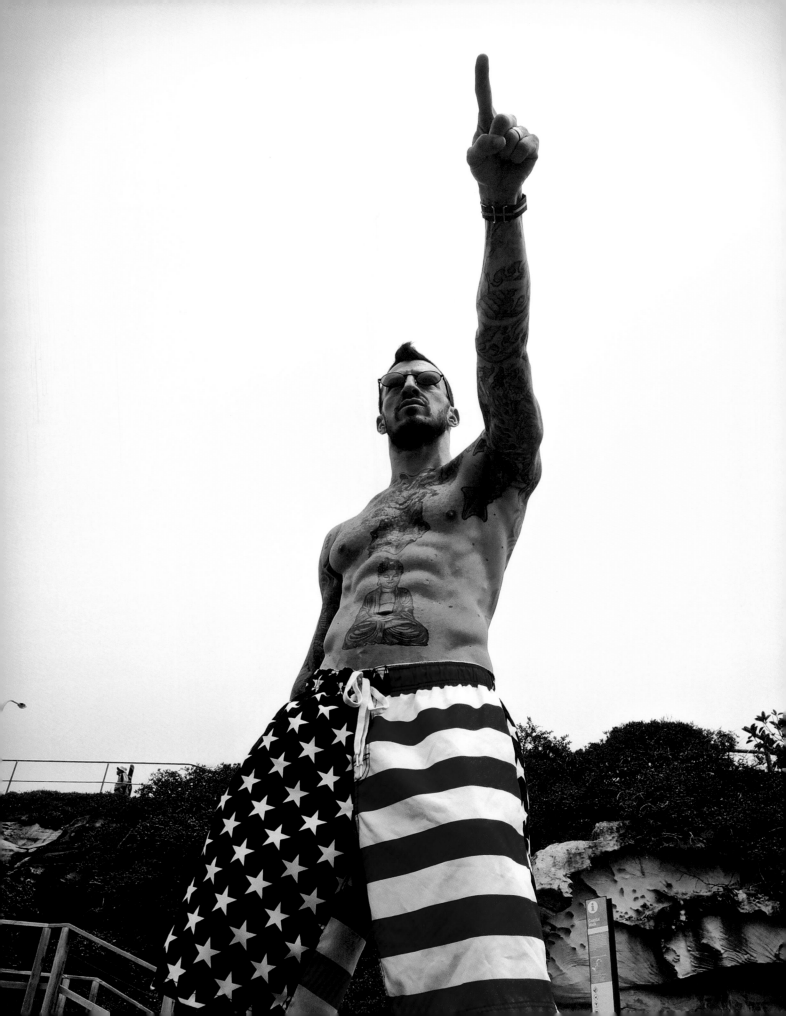

CHAPTER 11

MAKE AN EXECUTIVE DECISION

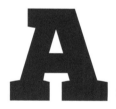re you ready to work hard?

Like much in life, if you want results, you must put forth effort. That is a good thing. There will always be voices in your head proclaiming reasons not to work out. Ignore them. Exercise is good! And it's crucial when your goal is a set of super Diamond-Cut Abs.

Training hard and consistently will be better for any individual than training half-assed and infrequently. This is not to say that everyone will get the exact same results if they put forth the same effort. I'm simply saying that there are no short cuts. Abs take time. You would never believe a gimmicky program called "7 Minute Marathoner" or "Couch To Black Belt in Karate", but for some reason we are very susceptible to misleading abs programs. Getting abs is like studying a martial art, or any other such discipline. It's a process that takes an indefinite amount of time and commitment. No matter how many years you do it, you continue your practice, not just to improve and maintain, but because it's a part of you.

When it comes to fitness, you choose your level of involvement. It's beautiful… the outcome rests solely on your individual effort. Absolutely no gym or equipment is necessary and no one can ever do the work for you. There is a special purity to that. Accountability. Empowerment. Self-improvement.

We can all find the time. No excuses.

In short, the choice to work out is yours and yours alone. You and only you are accountable for your actions. Make an executive decision and do it. Many things worth doing do not come easy.

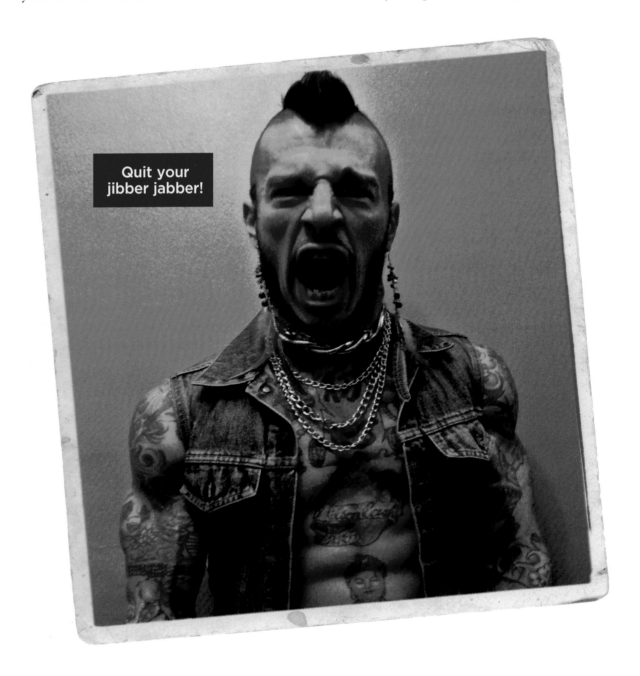

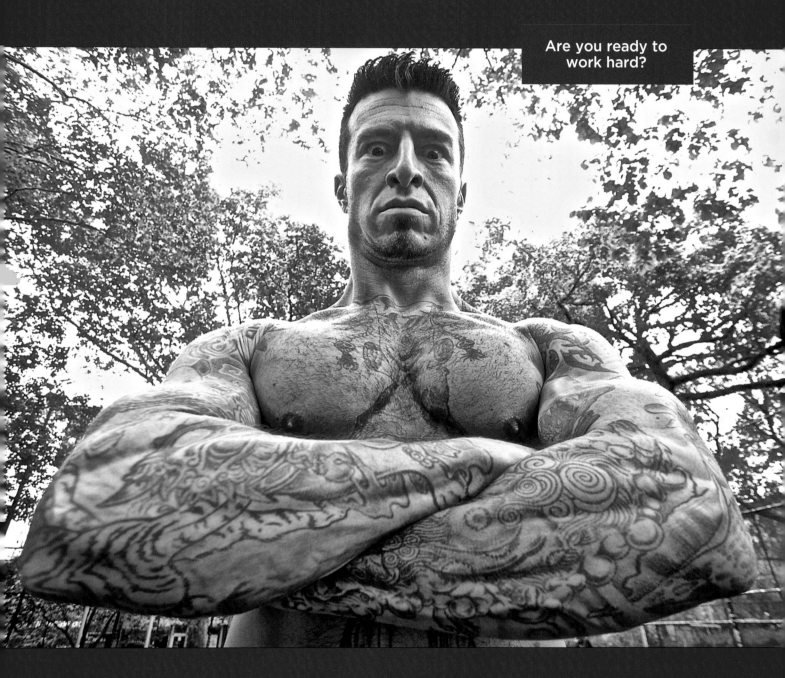

Are you ready to work hard?

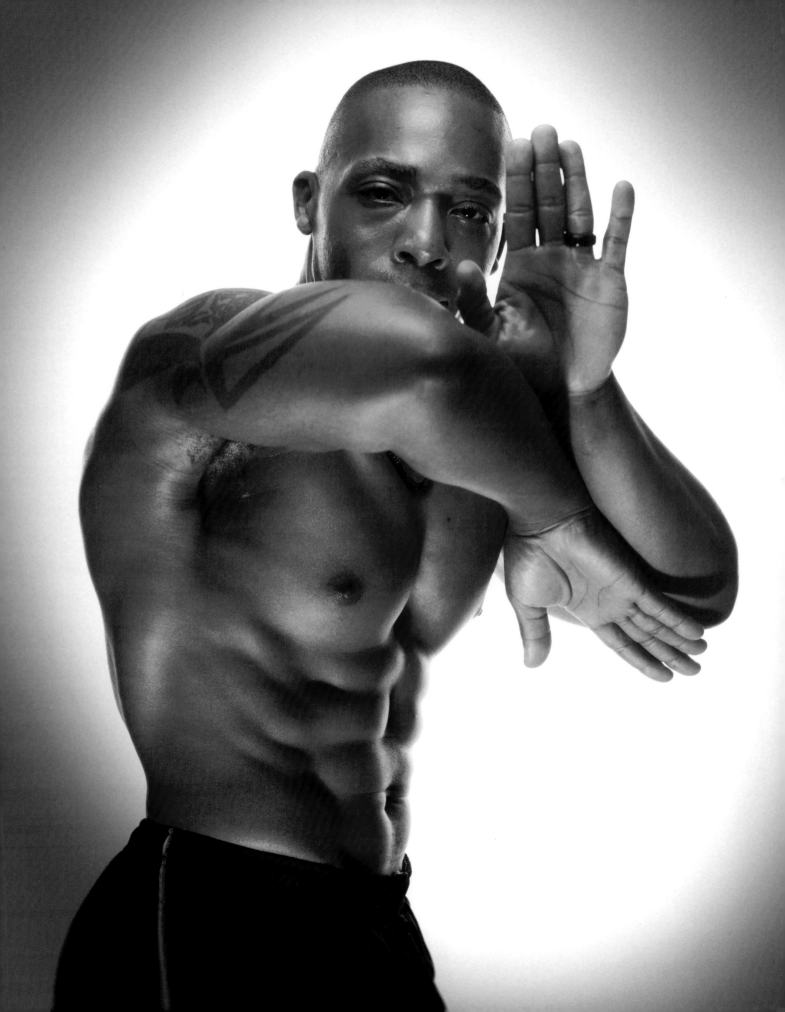

CHAPTER 12

FUNDAMENTALS OF ABDOMINAL STRENGTH TRAINING

Before embarking on our abs odyssey, there are certain principles we must discuss. Paying attention to them will help us to get the most from our journey. The following principles apply to every repetition of every exercise listed in this book.

Full Body Tension

The concept of full body tension will be easy for some people to grasp, and difficult for others. It means keeping some degree of rigidity throughout your entire body. Think back to the "core" or "powerhouse" we discussed in Chapter 2. I consider the core to include far more than just the abs and low back, but also the glutes, chest, upper back and even the shoulders—everything but the arms, legs and head. Yes, the exercises in this book focus on abs, even "isolating" them somewhat at times, but make no mistake: I believe you get your best gains from keeping your *entire body* engaged for the full range of motion of every single exercise. Don't ease up on the negative or rest on the bottom of a repetition. Keep everything tight. There's no true isolation, nor should there be. Full body tension makes you strong, anatomically aware and shredded. It helps facilitate everything.

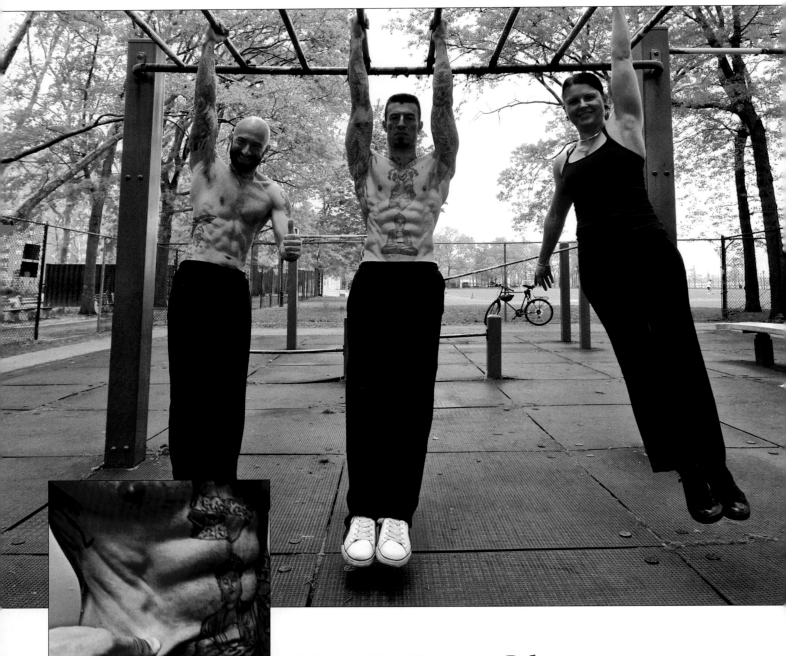

The Fallacy Of Spot Reduction

Training a specific part of the body will not lessen that area's fat in any way. Many people have a hard time accepting this but it is true. Yes, all exercise will reduce body fat to some degree (provided you don't counter it by eating more), but not necessarily in a predictable manner. That said, targeting a specific muscle or muscle group is sure to make it stronger, possibly bigger, just not necessarily lower in body fat. We can't predict from where the fat will be metabolized first, but we can make sure your abs are sculpted when the fat does come off.

Range Of Motion

If you want your muscles to get stronger and better defined, then perform the full range of motion (ROM) of every single exercise. Start at the very beginning position and, in a controlled fashion throughout, complete the full motion until the very ending position. This applies to most training in general, not just abs.

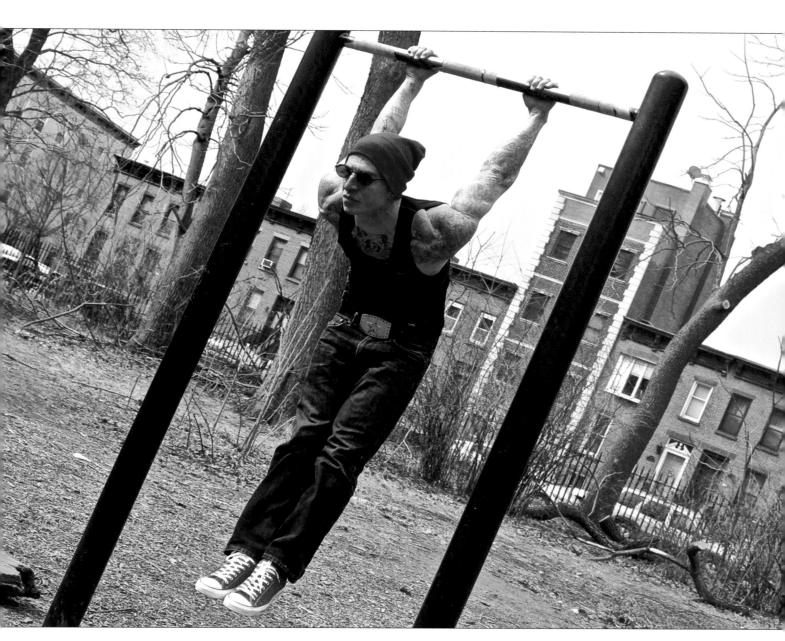

Complete Control

This refers to the attention and deliberation given to the movement of an exercise. Generally speaking, the speed should be unrushed, not necessarily "slow", but certainly not fast, and devoid of any bouncing or kipping. It's important to prioritize quality over quantity. The dynamic exercises in this book should all be performed with complete control, from start to finish, full ROM. Be certain to maintain control in the negatives and do not to rest at the bottom. Maintain tension instead! Do not use momentum. Obviously, isometric exercises don't have a range of motion, but complete control is still absolutely called for. In other words, no shaking, wavering, etc.

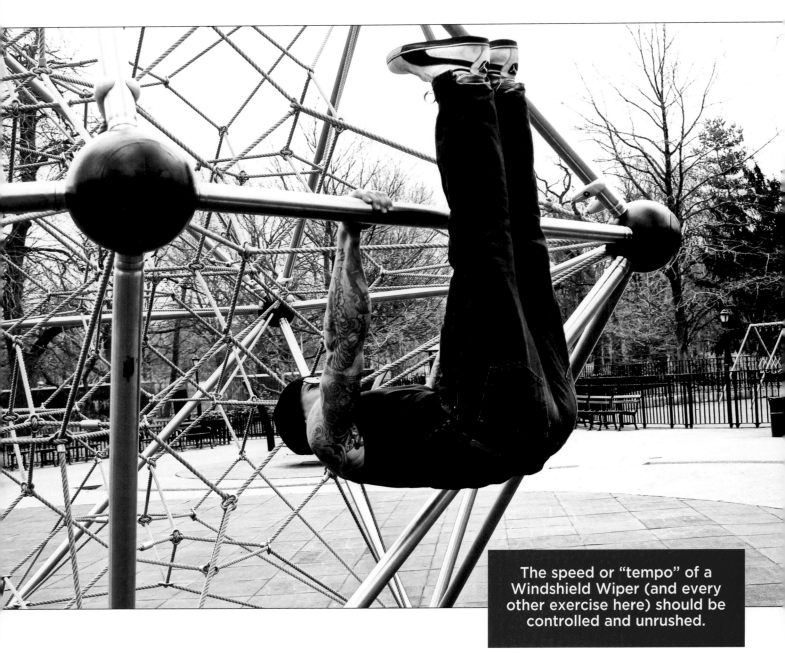

The speed or "tempo" of a Windshield Wiper (and every other exercise here) should be controlled and unrushed.

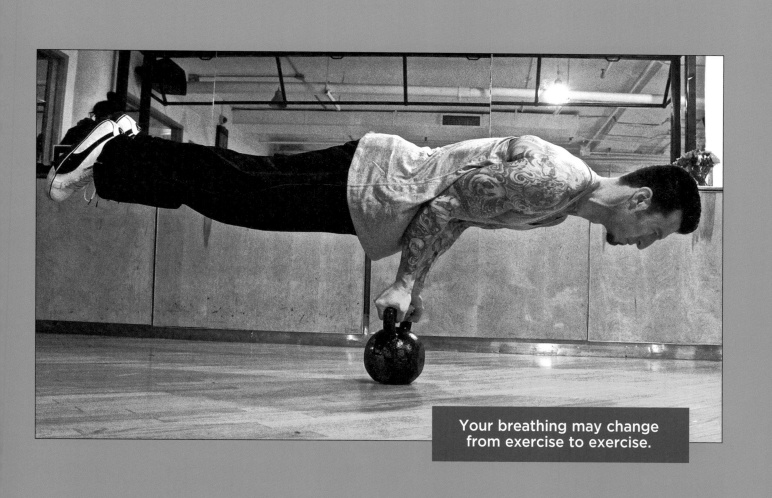

Your breathing may change from exercise to exercise.

Breathing

I do not have one general, blanket rule when it comes to breathing. In much of strength train-ing, we are taught to exhale when exerting and inhale when returning to the starting position of an exercise. This is a good rule of thumb but it does not apply to everything. Sometimes it feels good to hold your breath and create a "belly full of air" in order to maintain tension. Other times, you may prefer to keep tension and breathe very, very slowly through the nostrils. (This can be a great technique for isometrics.) Do what's comfortable to you. It may change from exercise to exercise… just don't forget to breathe altogether!

Progression

We are all on different fitness levels. In time, with consistent and appropriate training, we "progress" or make gains in our strength and skills. Manipulating leverage, performing harder exercises and doing higher reps are all ways of progressing. Depending on the exercise and your current fitness level, this can take weeks, months or years. I admit that it's fun to peak ahead, but if an exercise is truly out of your reach, it is unlikely you'll get much out of doing it. We want to do exercises that are challenging but do-able. Naturally, when an exercise ceases to be a challenge, then it's time to change it up.

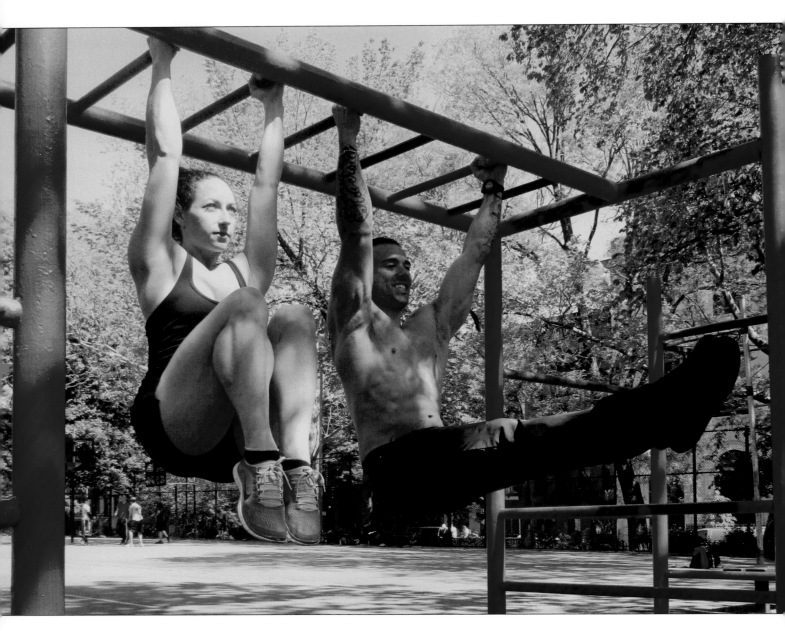

I may be biased here, but I think the notion of getting on a treadmill or pretend bike that doesn't go anywhere, with the goal of moving made-up numbers on a screen is bizarre. The "fat burning zone" on treadmills, as well as all the measurements and calculations, are as inauthentic as the machines themselves. The manufacturers want to sell treadmills to the gyms, which want to sell memberships to us, by adding a perceived value that they themselves fabricated. Get off the machine and actually move!

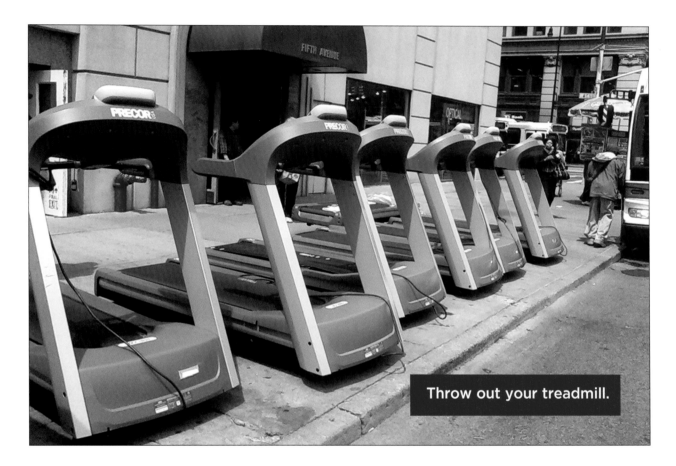

Throw out your treadmill.

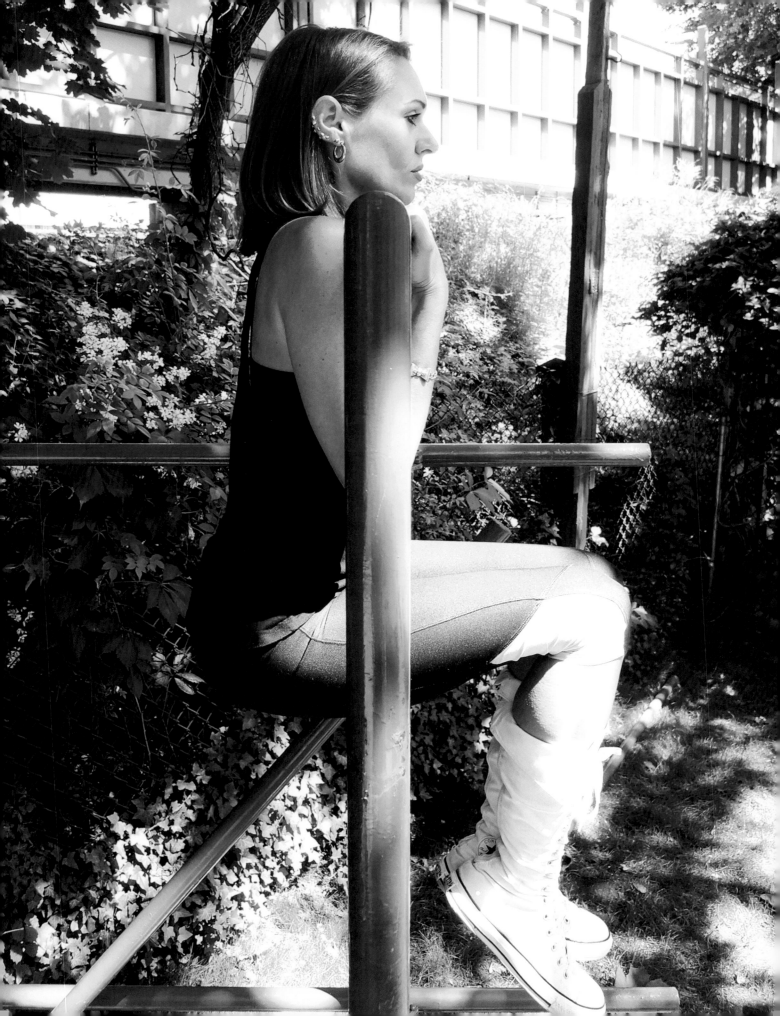

PART IV

THE EXERCISES

"Nothing will work unless you do."
—Maya Angelou

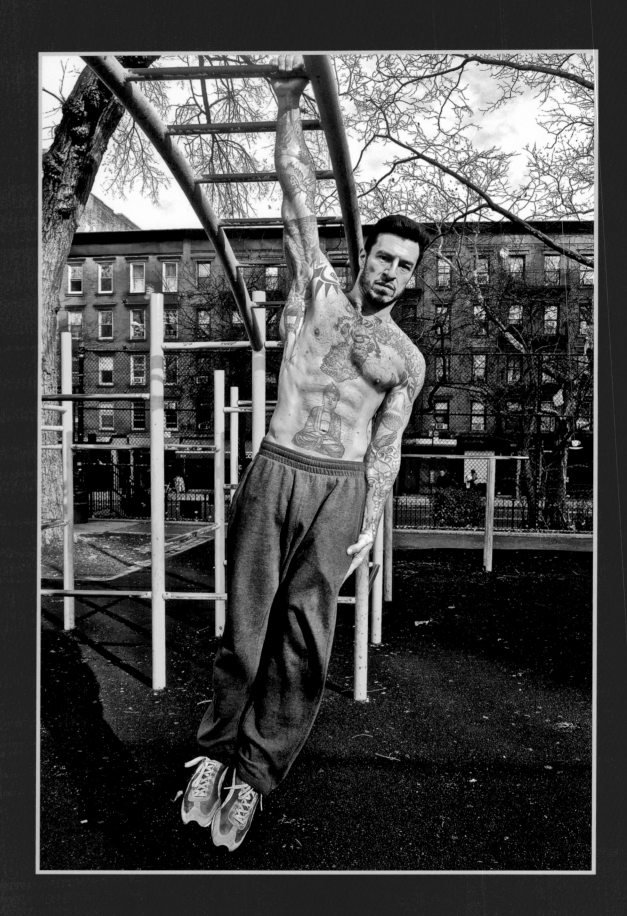

CHAPTER 14

"Danny, What Do You Do?"

I do a lot of things. This is a compilation of over fifty of the best abs and abs-related exercises I've ever done. They are broken down into Beginner, Intermediate and Advanced exercises. There is also a "CORE" Curriculum of basic strength training movements as training the abs only, while ignoring the rest of the body would be useless. Several supplemental stretches are included as well.

This is not a list of every abs exercise there is. Not even close. These are ones that have worked for me, as well as others at various stages in our respective training—they were not simply put together to make a book. I did not include exercises with which I do not have extensive experience. Every single one is relevant.

To be clear, you do not need any equipment at all to get world-class six-pack abs. Again, that figure is none. Zero. However, in the spirit of variety, as well as wanting to be as thorough as possible, I chose to also include several exercises that employ some minimalist gear, like a bench or pull-up bar. Real basic stuff.

The exercises are listed in a progressive order, but any "all purpose" absolute progression for all would be impossible to say. Sometimes the order is based on fluidity and consistency. The comparative difficulty may at times appear to move forward, backward, or even side-to-side. That's okay. All of our bodies move at different rates too. What you find easy, someone else may find difficult, and vice-versa. For that reason, all of the recommended Rep Ranges are rough estimates at best and may require weeks, months, even years to achieve. Be patient and respect your journey.

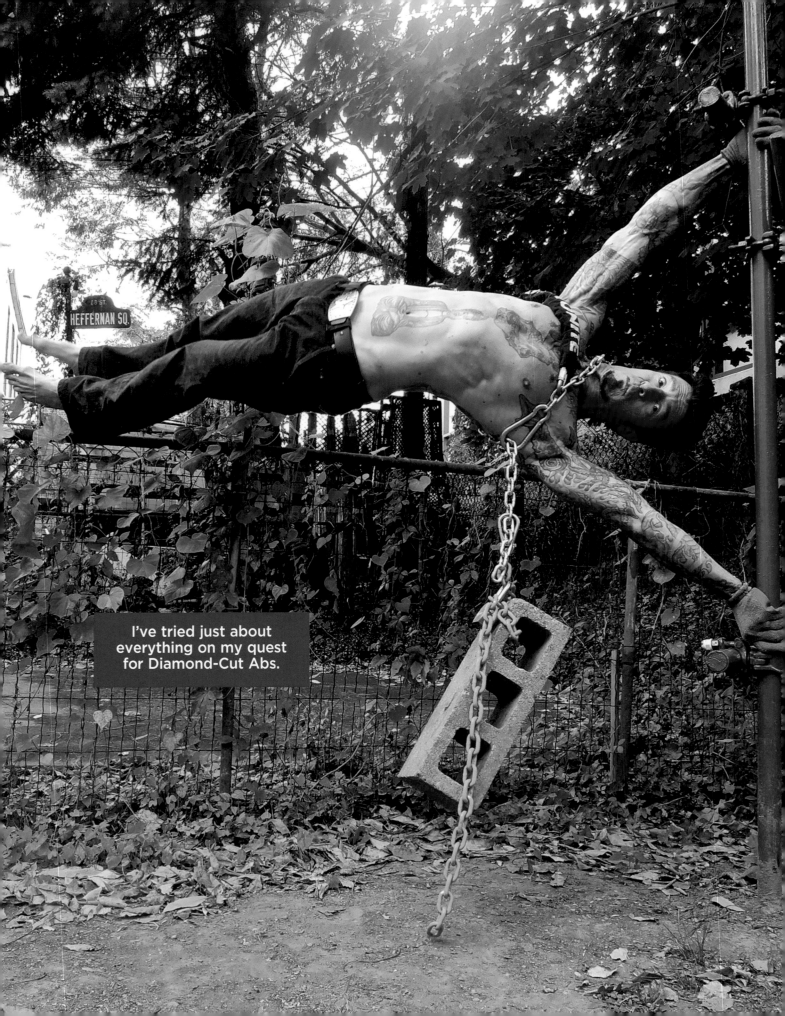

I've tried just about everything on my quest for Diamond-Cut Abs.

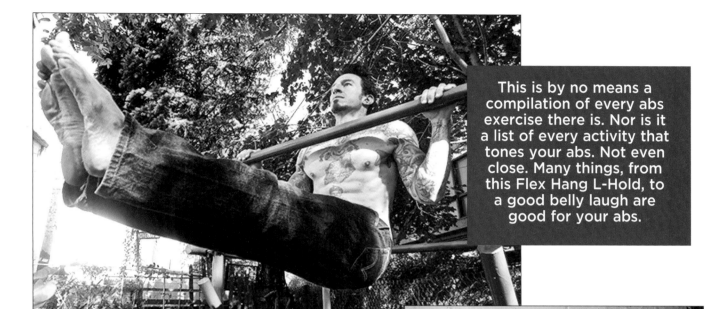

This is by no means a compilation of every abs exercise there is. Nor is it a list of every activity that tones your abs. Not even close. Many things, from this Flex Hang L-Hold, to a good belly laugh are good for your abs.

Keep tension throughout each exercise. Do not loosen up at the bottom position for any movements. Always be in control. If you are not in control you do not own the exercise. All of these exercises should be done with a full range of motion. The importance of form trumps any abstract rep goal. As far as reps are concerned, it is important to maintain a challenge. Just be aware that as the exercises increase in difficulty, rep ranges drop. Ultimately, twenty-five Sit-Ups will pose less of a challenge (and produce lower yields) than six or eight Dragon Flags. Refer back to Chapter 12 The Fundamentals Of Abdominal Strength Training for more on this subject.

There are a lot of exercises moving forward. I've also included trainer tips, common mistakes and some hard-earned advice. Use it all, but experiment and learn on your own too. Experience is the best teacher.

One more thing: While I absolutely encourage you to work on your favorite moves, it's still important to keep several exercises in rotation. (Luckily, the exercises herein have numerous variations!) The thing is, when your body gets used to doing the same things again and again and again, it will get very good at those things, but it's likely their effectiveness will diminish over time. It's important to mix it up to avoid plateaus, both physical and mental. Shock your system.

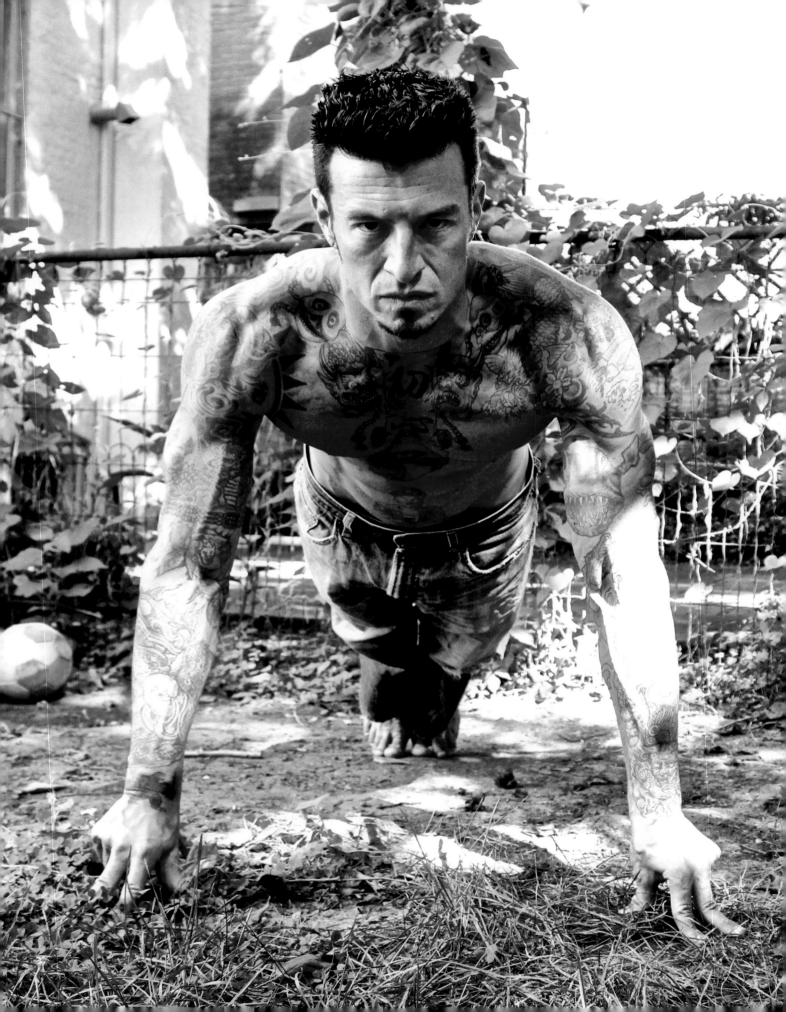

CHAPTER 15

CORE CURRICULUM

These exercises are important for strength, health and life. Ultimately, they will yield greater over-all gains than any abs-only program ever will. In fact, an abs workout should only be practiced in addition to, *not instead of*, a complete full-body program. These exercises train everything. It's as simple as squat, push, pull.

These CORE Curriculum exercises and their unlimited variations will provide the foundation for a lifetime of strength training; I deliberately kept it basic. Just remember, no matter how chiseled your six-pack looks, you're not strong until you are comfortable at these exercises, which all work your abs in their own right.

SQUAT

Squats are probably the most functional exercise there is. Oddly, those who are brand new to exercise (or have been sedentary for a long time) sometimes feel that Squats are "unnatural". This is often because many folks have spent years deconditioning themselves to what is one of the oldest movement patterns in our DNA. Squats are, in fact, very natural.

Begin by standing with your feet flat on the ground. I prefer doing Squats barefoot, as that helps me establish a better connection with my surroundings, but that's just a personal preference. A solid footing is key. Start putting you butt out behind you, as if about to sit down, making sure to bend at both the knee and the hip. Get as low as your mobility will allow, while keeping you chest up. Now press your heels through the ground and push your hips forward so you return to a standing position. Squats work your legs, low back and abs, as well as your neurological and cardiovascular systems.

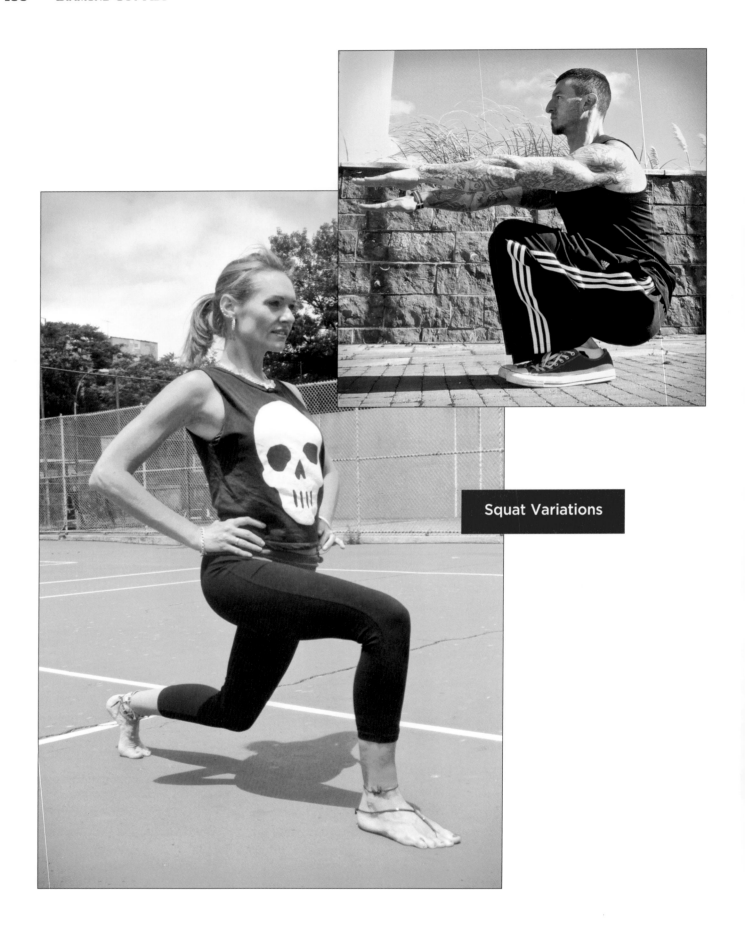

Squat Variations

There are unlimited variations of the Squat, from merely sitting down and standing up, to lunges, to advanced single-legged versions, to name just a few.

Trainer Talk: It's important to get your hips beneath you knees at the bottom of the repetition. Some variations are harder to get low than others and some people are more flexible than others. Mobility comes in time. Stay the course.

Rep Range: Forty bodyweight squats in a row is a solid baseline.

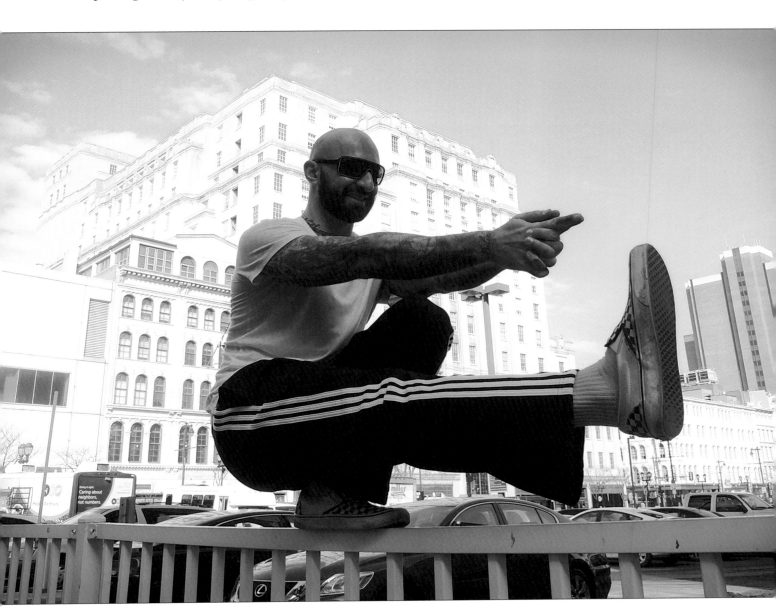

PUSH-UP

Push-Ups are the ultimate upper body exercise. Although the primary movers are the pectorals and triceps, a strong core, along with powerful shoulders and lats, are key. Place your hands on the ground, just wider than your shoulders, with your feet together and your body straight. Keep you chin up. Bend at the elbows and lower your chest down until it almost touches the ground beneath you. Now press yourself back up and lock out at the elbows. That is one rep.

Because women tend to be less naturally endowed toward upper body strength than men, Knee Push-ups, a variation where the hands and knees are placed on the ground, rather than the hands and feet, can be a viable starting point. This changes the length of the body, thus adjusting the leverage. Additionally, altering inclines, changing the distance between hands or feet, even incorporating grip challenges (fingertip, knuckles , etc.) make the Push-Up unbelievable scalable.

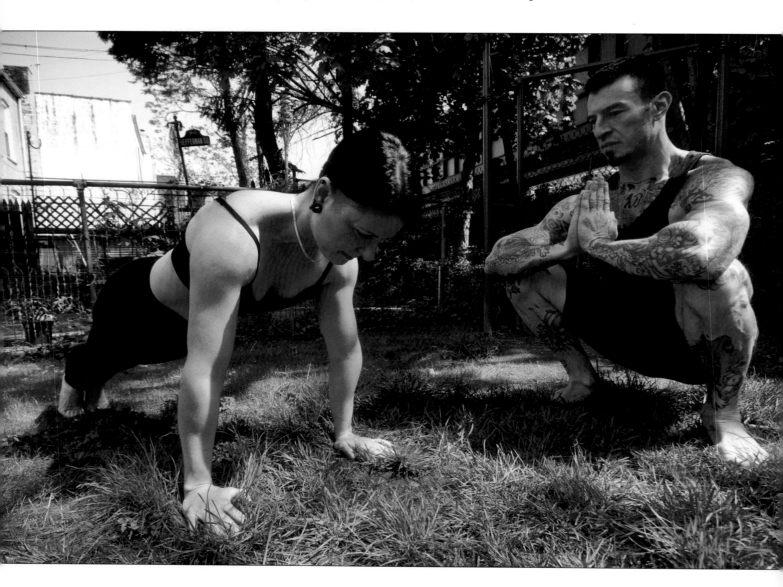

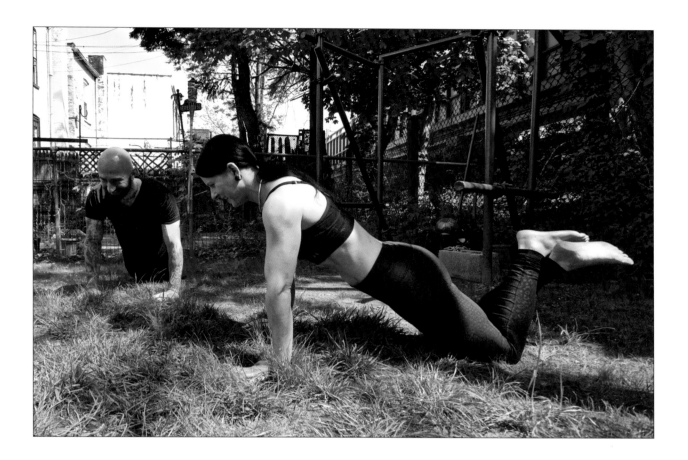

Trainer Talk: Many exercises that are not technically "Push-ups" incorporate similar movement patterns and emphasize the same muscle groups. Examples include Dips, Handstand Pushups, Overhead Presses and more. They all involve an upper body pressing motion.

Rep Range: 30 Push-ups is a solid starting point for men. 30 Knee Push-Ups for women.

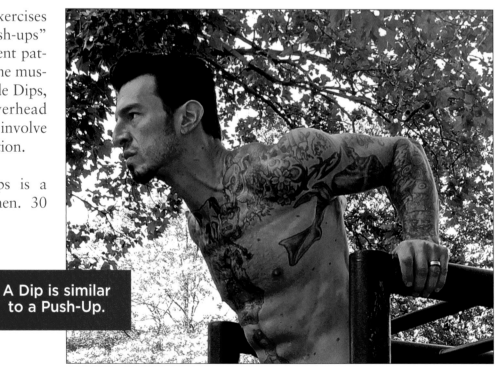

A Dip is similar to a Push-Up.

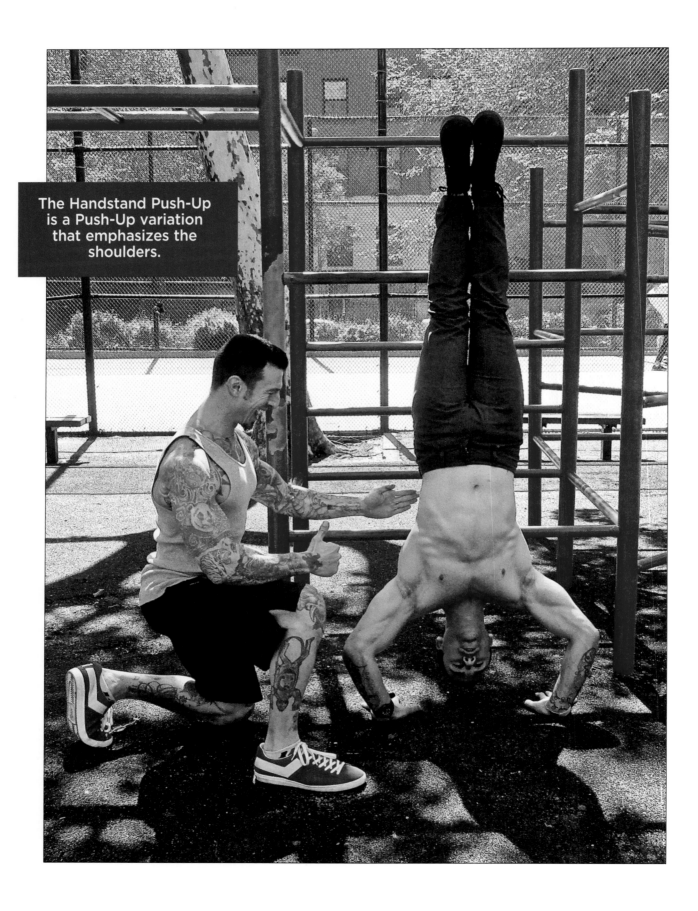

The Handstand Push-Up is a Push-Up variation that emphasizes the shoulders.

PULL-UP

I love Pull-Ups. 'Nuff said.

Start by hanging from the bar with your shoulder blades retracted. Be mentally inside every muscle in your body. Pull the bar towards your sternum until your chin goes over the bar. Now lower your body down into a hang again. That is one rep.

Though technically a Pull-Up means an overhand grip, "Chin-Ups", their underhanded counterpart, as well as parallel and switch grips, are all official in my book.

Like the Push-Up, females (and many males) may initially be inclined to a slight variation. The Australian Pull-Up (or Body Row) is an excellent alternative. With your heels on the ground and your body straight, hang from a horizontal bar of approximately waist height. Maintain a straight line from the shoulder to the hip to the heel. It should look like an upside-down Push-Up. Now, with your shoulder blades back, pull the bar toward your chest until the arms are flexed past 90 degrees at the elbow. Slowly return to the starting position. That is one rep.

Trainer Talk: If Pull-Ups prove difficult for beginners, numerous regressions exist besides the Australian Pull-Up. These include assisted Pull-Ups, partial Pull-Ups and slow negatives. By the same token, there are infinite progressions as well. Everything from odd-surface grips to Muscle-Ups are advanced.

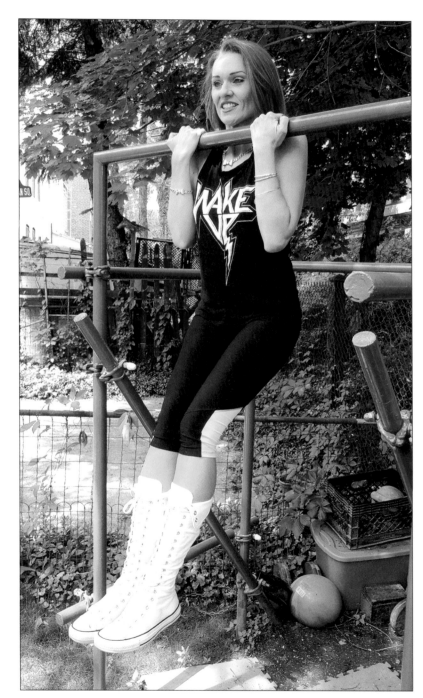

Rep Range: Ten reps is solid for men. Ten Australian Pull-Ups for the ladies.

Pull-Up Variations

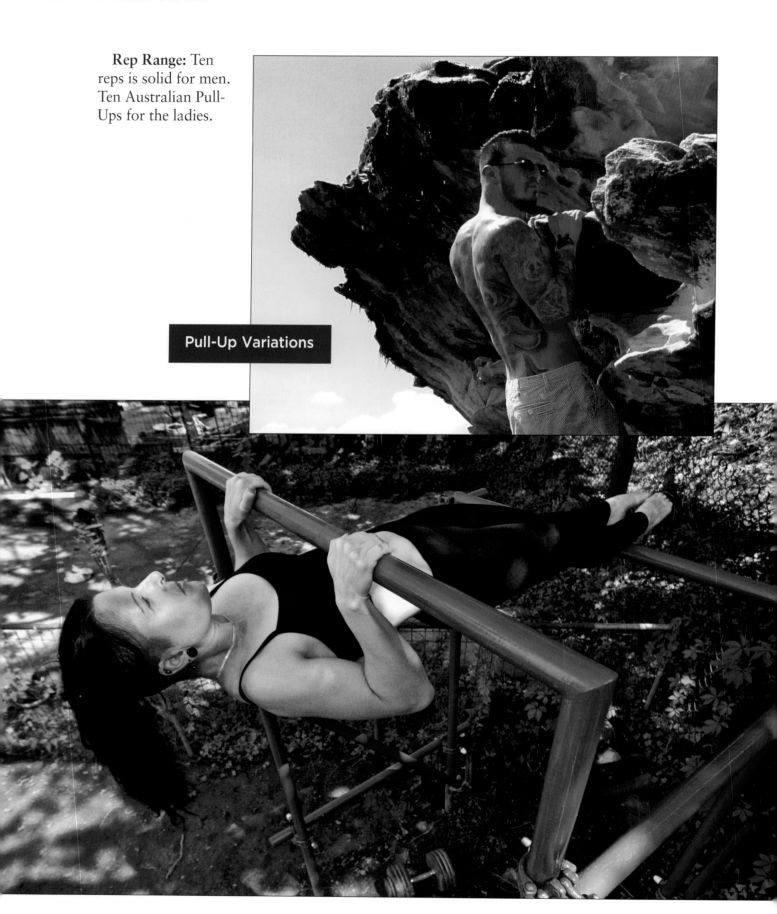

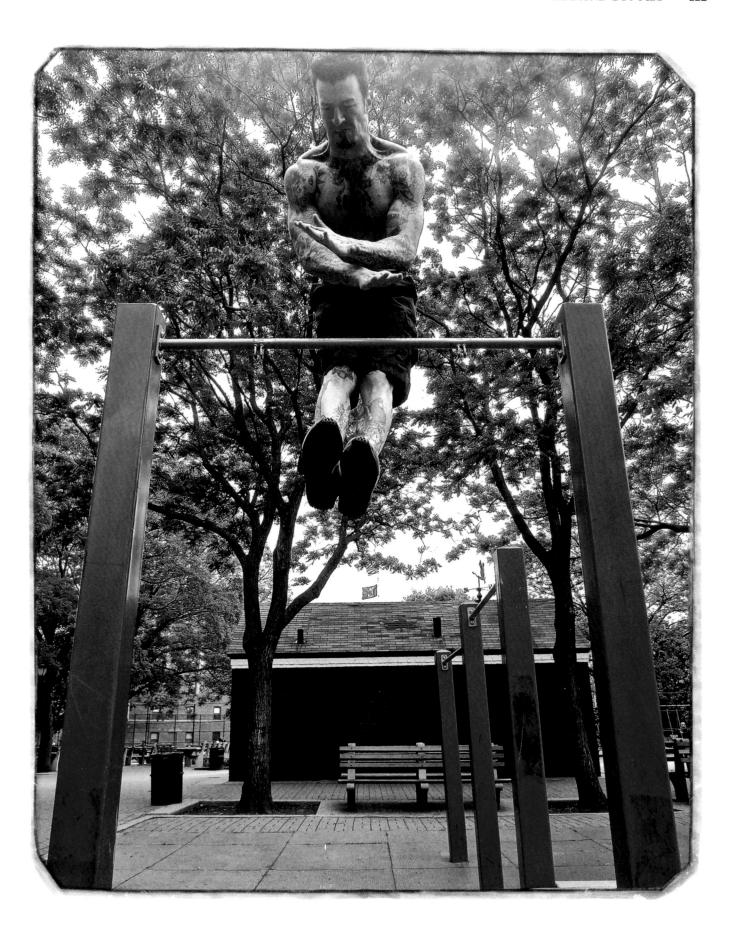

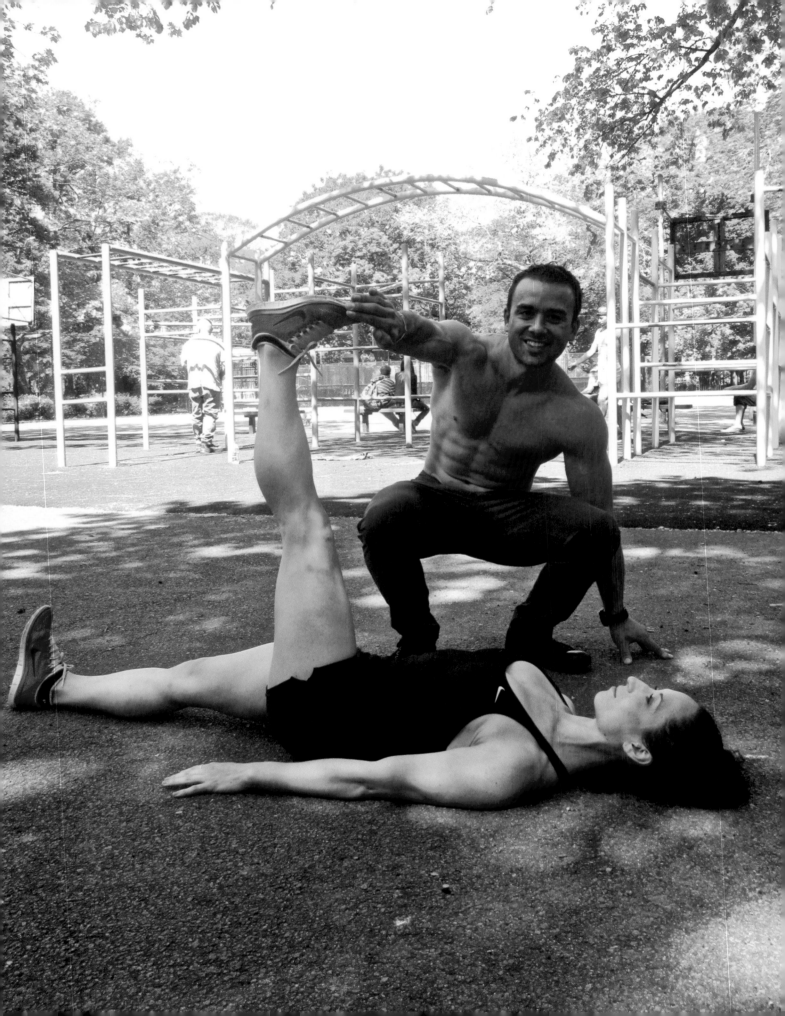

CHAPTER 16

BEGINNER ABS

When you begin to train your abs, you may not know where to start. As we discussed in Chapter 2, there is no real "upper" or "lower" abs (the rectus abdominis is one muscle), however I will refer to these terms from time to time, as some exercises place different emphasis than others. Beginners sometimes find these cues helpful. When I say "upper" (as in Sit-Ups for example), I mean the location of the top two to four cubes of a six-pack. When I say "lower" (as in Leg Raises), I'm referring to the area starting around the belly button, down to the hips and below the waist. It goes without saying that both Sit-Ups and Leg Raises employ the entirety of your abdominals for stability and strength. The terms "upper" and "lower" abs refer to emphasis not isolation.

Please consider all recommended rep ranges with a grain of salt. They are loose guidelines at best. It may take beginners 3-6 months, or years in some cases, to move onto harder exercises, even within the Beginner Abs category. Be patient. Take as much recovery time as you need between sets. Respect the journey.

You will not just get stronger when you begin a program, you will also start to establish pathways within your nervous system, as your body learns the movement patterns. A great deal of strength is neurological. It cannot be separated. Good luck!

FULL BODY TENSION DRILL

For any of this to work, you must be aware of your body. This drill is appropriate for every uninjured individual of any fitness level, from the novice to the elite, even if you've never worked out before. Start by standing up, feet flat on the floor, shoulder width apart. There should be an invisible plumb line from your shoulder, to your hip, down to your heel. Press your feet into the floor. Wiggle your toes, feel your heels, use your feet to grip the ground beneath you. Tighten your legs and butt. Your abs and back. Make a fist. Squeeze your hands and arms. Everything. Try to focus on each muscle as you feel it activate. This is an isometric drill, meaning your muscles are in a fixed position rather than going through a range of motion. Hold it and release. Take several deep breaths. Shake your hands and feet. Repeat as many times as you feel appropriate.

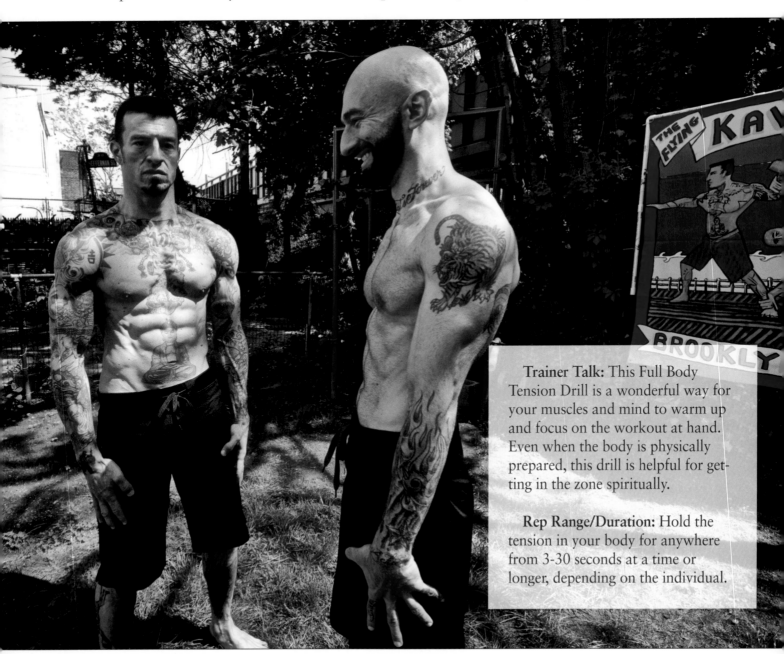

Trainer Talk: This Full Body Tension Drill is a wonderful way for your muscles and mind to warm up and focus on the workout at hand. Even when the body is physically prepared, this drill is helpful for getting in the zone spiritually.

Rep Range/Duration: Hold the tension in your body for anywhere from 3-30 seconds at a time or longer, depending on the individual.

PLANK

The Plank has its roots in yoga but has been widely adapted into all types of strength training. Like the Full Body Tension Drill, it's an isometric exercise. Also like the Full Body Tension Drill, it's a great starting point. Begin in a horizontal position on the ground. Place your feet together, with your forearms on the floor, elbow to wrist. The body should be straight. Tense the entire body including the abs, glutes, arms and legs. Engage everything.

The Plank can also be performed with the arms extended like the top of a Push-Up or by placing the arms on an elevated surface, hence shortening the length of the body. Conversely, the plank can be progressed by elevating the feet.

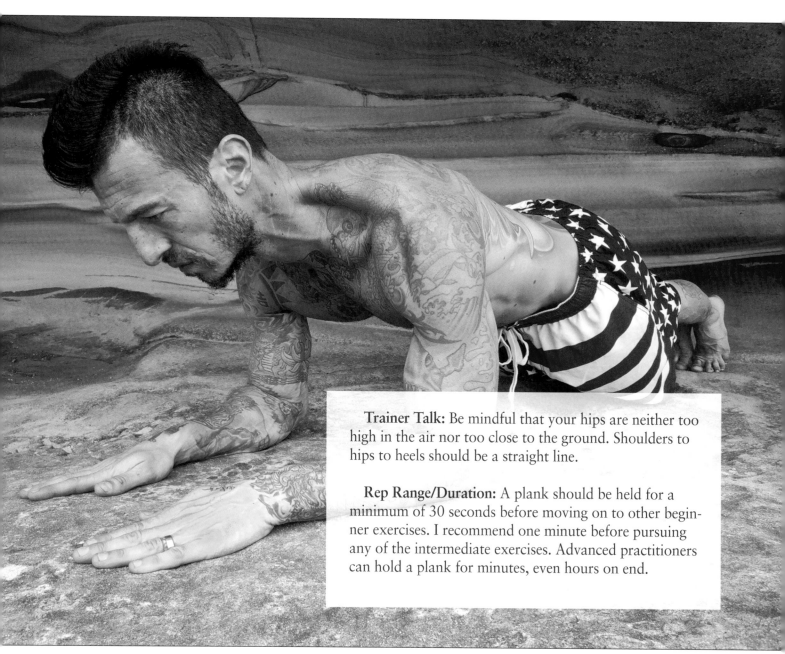

Trainer Talk: Be mindful that your hips are neither too high in the air nor too close to the ground. Shoulders to hips to heels should be a straight line.

Rep Range/Duration: A plank should be held for a minimum of 30 seconds before moving on to other beginner exercises. I recommend one minute before pursuing any of the intermediate exercises. Advanced practitioners can hold a plank for minutes, even hours on end.

SIDE PLANK

The Side Plank is a variation of the classic Plank that places extra emphasis on the obliques and the entire lateral chain. I like going into the Side Plank from the top of a Push-Up position. From that top position, pivot your body so that one hand is on the ground directly under the shoulder with your feet together and your side facing the floor beneath you. Keep tension throughout your entire body. Make sure you train each side evenly.

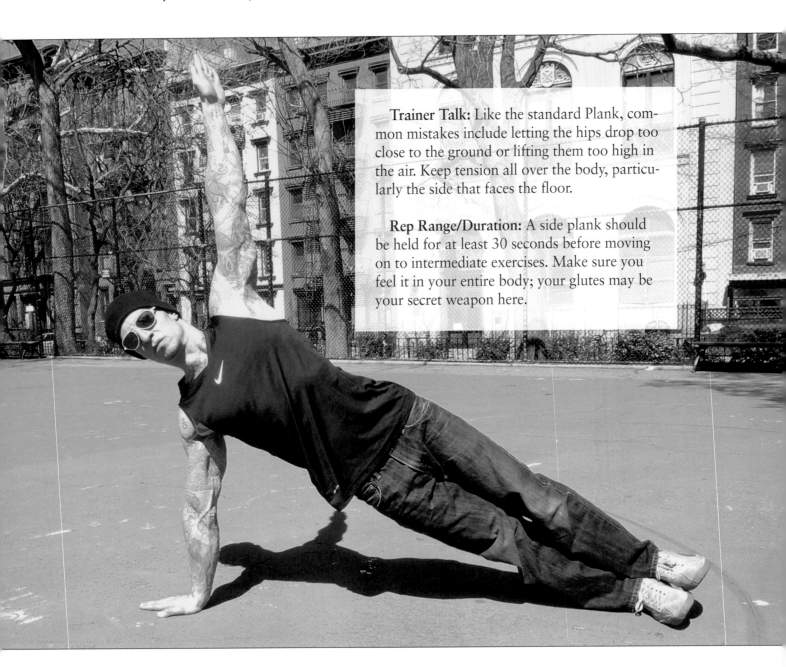

Trainer Talk: Like the standard Plank, common mistakes include letting the hips drop too close to the ground or lifting them too high in the air. Keep tension all over the body, particularly the side that faces the floor.

Rep Range/Duration: A side plank should be held for at least 30 seconds before moving on to intermediate exercises. Make sure you feel it in your entire body; your glutes may be your secret weapon here.

LYING SINGLE LEG RAISE

To perform a Lying Single Leg Raise, lie on the ground with your palms flat. Without pressing into the ground, bring one leg straight up so it's perpendicular to the floor. Now lower it all the way down, then repeat on the other side. This exercise is best suited to someone new to training their abs. It can be regressed by bending the knee and shortening the length of the moving leg. A slight kink in either knee may be unavoidable at the top position, depending on individual hamstring flexibility.

Trainer Talk: To progress, try raising the grounded leg up, as the other comes down, rather than waiting until it returns to the starting position. This "flutter kick" movement is a step on their path toward Straight Leg Raises and ultimately, all hanging abs.

Rep Range: After you can perform 2-3 sets of 15 per leg, move on to Lying Bent Knee Raises.

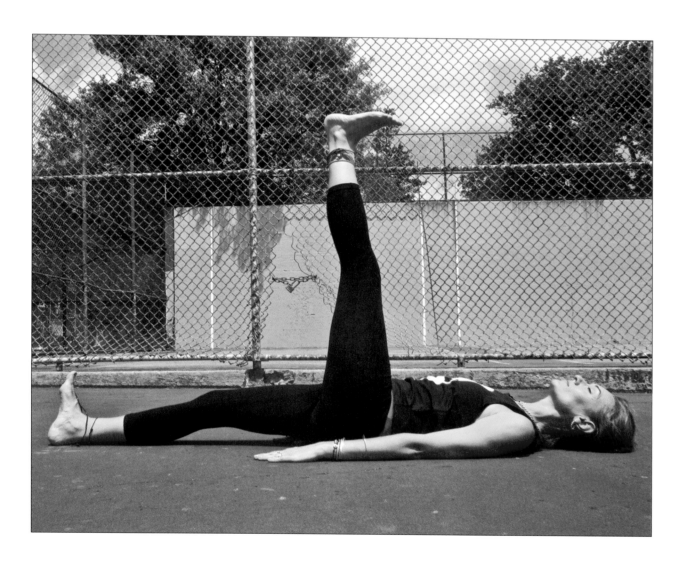

LYING BENT KNEE LEG RAISE

The Lying Bent Knee Raise picks up where the Single Leg Raise leaves off. Start by lying on the ground, palms down, legs together. Maintain a bend in the knees. The more obtuse the angle of the bend, the more challenging the exercise is. Now contract your abs to bring your legs up off the ground simultaneously. The angle of flexion at the knee should not change as your legs go up and your legs should remain together. Lower them down to the starting position and repeat. Once you are comfortable, try them without letting your heels touch the ground at the bottom of the motion.

Lying Bent Knee Raises can also be performed on an incline to increase the resistance. The exercise gets more challenging as the incline increases.

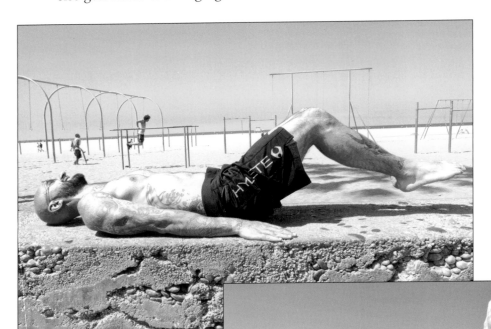

Trainer Talk: This exercise is a great pre-cursor to all hanging knee raises. Get good at it!

Rep Range: Become comfortable performing 3 sets of 15-20 reps before moving onto the bar.

LYING KNEE TUCK

This exercise is very similar to Lying Bent Knee Leg Raises. The main distinction is that instead of lifting the leg up and "reverse" crunching the lower body, think of drawing the knees toward the chest in a smooth, continuous motion. Bring your knees as high up toward your chest as your range of motion will allow. Now extend your legs out until they're totally straight, almost parallel to the ground, but do not let your heels touch the ground. Repeat.

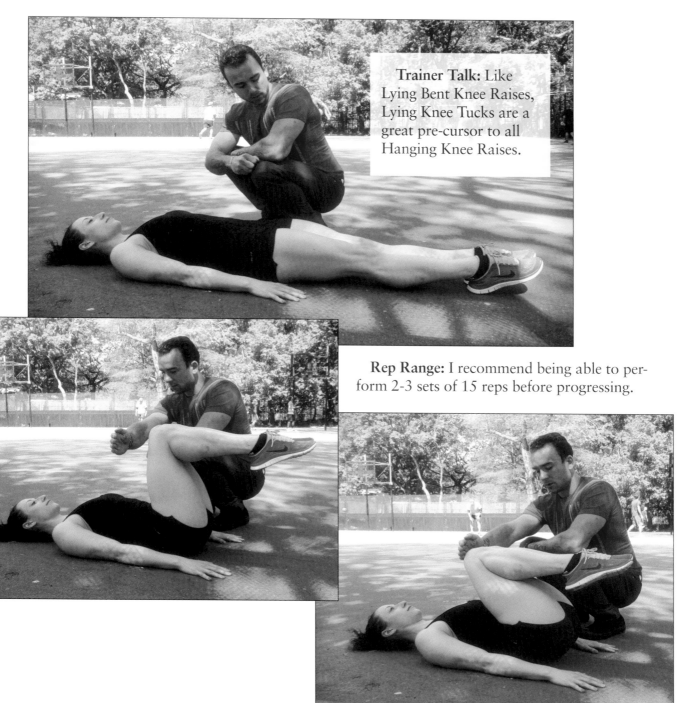

Trainer Talk: Like Lying Bent Knee Raises, Lying Knee Tucks are a great pre-cursor to all Hanging Knee Raises.

Rep Range: I recommend being able to perform 2-3 sets of 15 reps before progressing.

SIT-UP

Folks from my generation are well acquainted with Sit-Ups. They are every bit as much a calisthenics cornerstone as Squats and Push-Ups. To perform a Sit-Up, lie on the ground with your knees up. Keep both feet flat on the floor. I prefer keeping my arms crossed over my chest, but there are other popular hand positions, including hands behind head. Squeeze with your abs until your upper body comes all the way up toward your knees, into a sitting up, as the name implies. Hold the top position for a breath, fully tense and in complete control, then lower back down and repeat. It may be helpful at the beginning to stabilize your feet under an object or with a partner.

Sit-ups have been decried as being bad for your neck and back. Anything has the potential to be dangerous. I can fall down walking, but walking is not bad for you. When doing Sit-Ups, be certain you're initiating the movement with your abs and take care not to shrug your shoulders. A mat can also be useful.

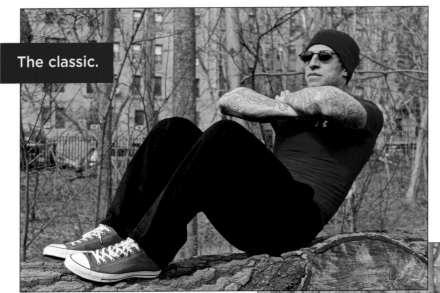

The classic.

Trainer Talk: Sit-ups can be modified by adding a twist at the top of the movement, thus further recruiting the obliques.

Rep Range: When you can do 3 sets of 20 controlled, quality sit-ups, you can start experimenting with Advanced Sit-Ups.

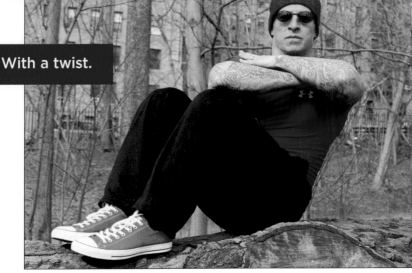

With a twist.

MODIFIED SIDE JACKKNIFE

The Modified Side Jackknife is designed for beginners to target their obliques. Performing Modified Side Jackknives is useful to those new to training their abs, although in time, they can be phased out in favor of classic Side Jackknife.

Start out by lying on your right side with your legs together and both knees bent. Keep your right arm close to your body and place your left hand behind your ear, bending at the left elbow. Squeeze your obliques to bring your top leg and your torso together, touching the knee to elbow. Be certain to get the upper body off the floor, not just the head and neck. Finish your set and repeat on the other side. To progress, you can try bending less and less at the knees. This will make the exercise more challenging by using your own leverage against you.

Trainer Talk: I find it helpful to reach over with the opposite hand and feel those obliques work. In other words, when contracting your left side, reach over with your right hand. This will provide a physical cue for the appropriate muscles.

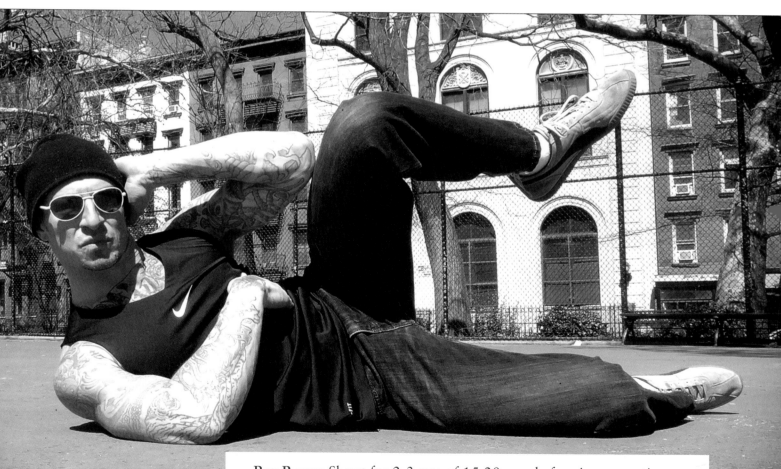

Rep Range: Shoot for 2-3 sets of 15-20 reps before incorporating standard, unmodified Side Jackknives into your program.

CROSSOVER

The Crossover fuses the elements of the Sit-Up and the Modified Side Jackknife. Start out by lying on the ground with your knees up and feet flat. Cross your left leg over your right, like a figure 4, with your ankle close to your knee and your knee away from your torso. Now bring your right hand behind your head and twist your right elbow to your left knee, without moving the knee. Complete your set and repeat on the other side.

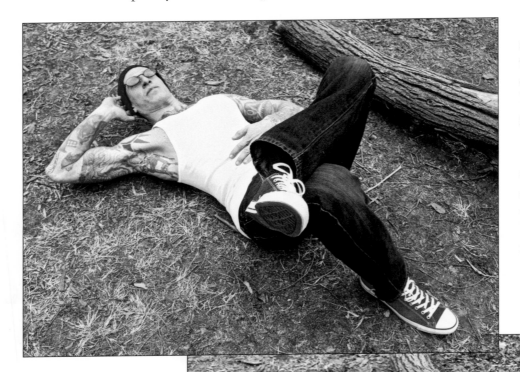

Trainer Talk: Make sure to rotate your trunk, not just move the elbow. The shoulder blade must come off the ground.

Rep Range: Beginners should work towards a solid 3 sets of 15-20 on each side in order to build a foundation for more challenging moves.

I like to keep the "non-crossing over" hand right on my abs so I can feel them working.

BICYCLE

The Bicycle adds the "lower" abs to the Crossover. Lie down with your hips and knees bent to ninety degrees each, shins parallel to the ground. Bring your left shoulder off the ground and twist to the right, as you simultaneously bring your right knee toward your left elbow. Repeat on the other side in a continuous motion. This "pedaling" of the lower body is said to resemble the act of riding a bicycle.

Trainer Talk: Make sure to rotate your trunk, not just move the elbow toward the knee. Be mindful to squeeze from your abs not your neck.

Rep Range: A fluid, non-stop 50 (alternating 1 rep per side smoothly) is a good short term goal. Even with control and deliberation, Bicycles can go by quickly so be mindful not to rush. Once you have confidence and control of this exercise, it can be eliminated altogether in favor of lower reps of more advanced exercises, like Hanging Knee Raises, for example.

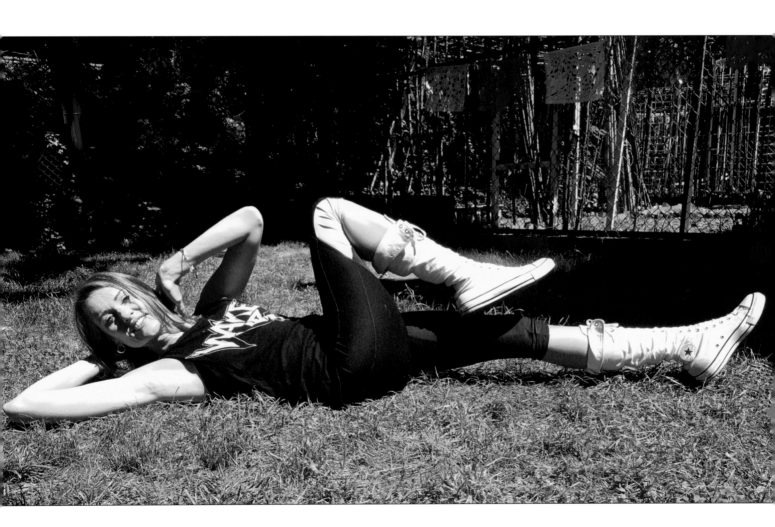

STRAIGHT ARM/STRAIGHT LEG CROSSOVER

You can progress the Standard Crossover to a more difficult variation simply by lengthening your body, which increases your leverage and in turn, resistance. To do so, instead of bending at elbow and knee, simply straighten out your arms and legs. There's not much more to it.

Start by lying on your back, with your left arm extended and your hand overhead. Now squeeze from the abs to bring your shoulder blade off the ground as you simultaneously raise your right leg. Twist at the trunk so that the elbow meets the opposite knee. Return to the starting position. Make sure that you are squeezing with you abs, not leading with your neck or using momentum. Train both sides equally.

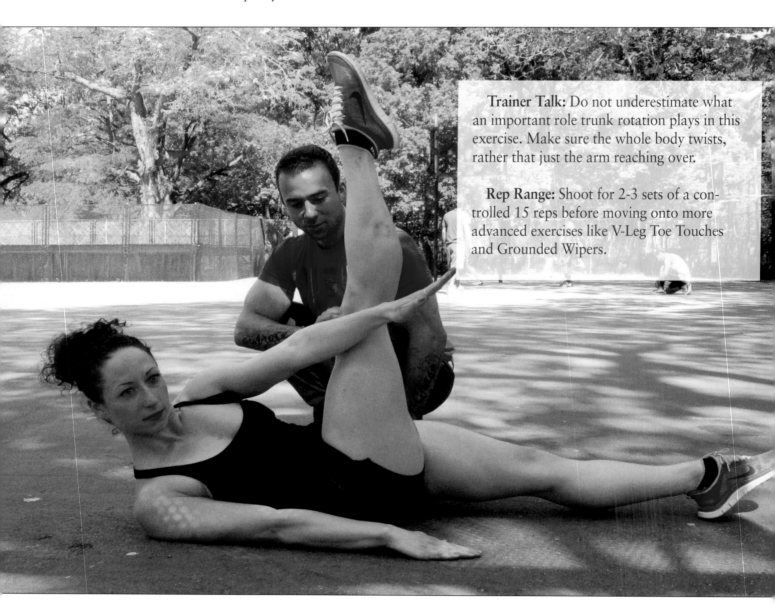

Trainer Talk: Do not underestimate what an important role trunk rotation plays in this exercise. Make sure the whole body twists, rather that just the arm reaching over.

Rep Range: Shoot for 2-3 sets of a controlled 15 reps before moving onto more advanced exercises like V-Leg Toe Touches and Grounded Wipers.

V-LEG TOE TOUCH

This is a nice, simple exercise designed to work all the superficial muscles of the abs. Begin by lying on your back with legs straight up and spread in a "V" formation. Keeping your hands straight overhead, use your abs to squeeze and twist your trunk so that your right hand points toward your left foot. Even if you cannot touch your foot, go as far as your range of motion will allow. Slowly return to the starting position. Then repeat on the other side.

Trainer Talk: I recommend keeping the knees unlocked when the legs are extended. This keeps the focus on the abs doing the work, not the legs.

Rep Range: When you can perform more than 30 in a row, alternating left and right, and feel like you could do it all day, then you're on your way to Intermediate Abs!

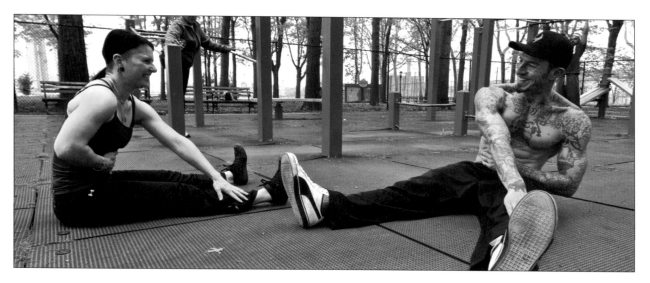

Why No Crunches?

I made an executive decision not to include Crunches on my list of exercises. Although I don't think they are as inherently evil as the detractors say, I cannot endorse them either. My problem with Crunches is not the potential neck strain often associated with poor form. (I don't like to fall victim to the fear-mongering techniques of the fitness world.) Rather, my issue is that by design, the Crunch deliberately discourages the connection between different parts of the body—parts that are intended to function harmoniously. That's not my style.

But like many beginners, I loved Crunches as a youth. My relationship with them lasted far too long, as most young romances do. So learn from my mistakes or experiment for yourself. It's up to you, but I believe that every single exercise in this book will yield far greater gains.

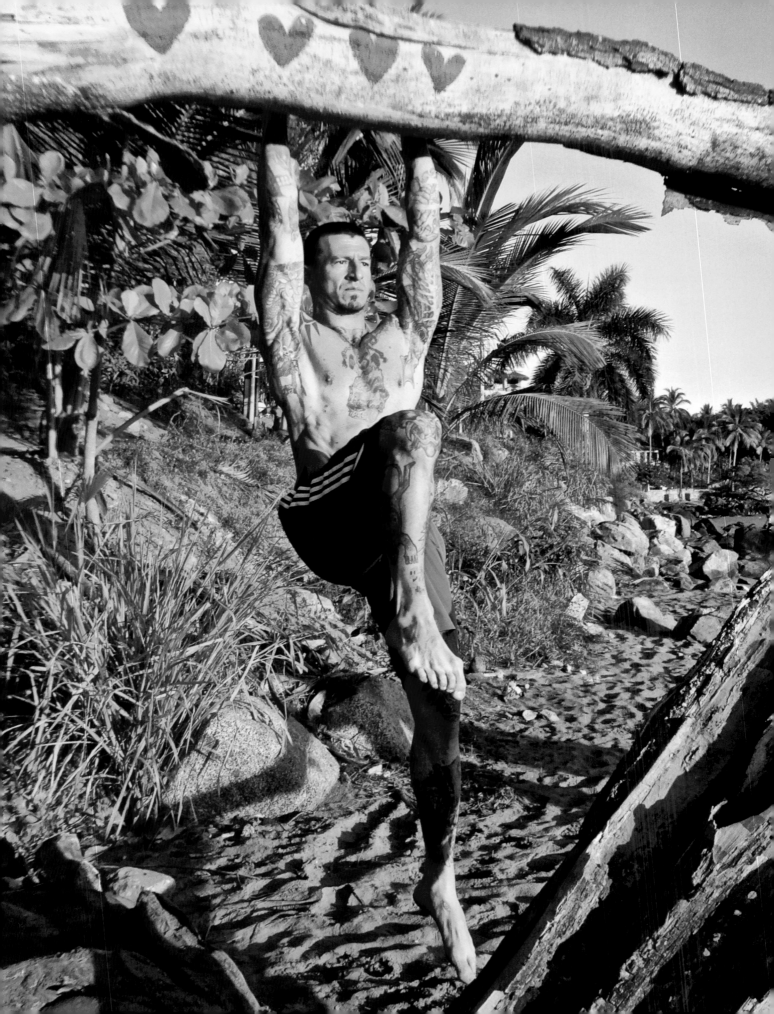

INTERMEDIATE ABS

As we advance past Beginner Abs, there will be less and less references to "upper" and "lower" abs. Like we discussed earlier, we want the entire abs (and body) to work together to get strong! Thinking in terms of separation becomes less relevant after the very beginning stage.

As with Beginner Abs exercises, the following rep ranges are simply guidelines and aim to serve only as an approximation. The exercises in this chapter can (and should) be done for months, even years if necessary, before moving onto Advanced Abs.

UNSTABLE PLANK

No matter how far along you progress on your abs odyssey, I believe that the timeless Plank should always have a place in your voyage. A fun way to add an extra challenge is to bring instability into the mix.

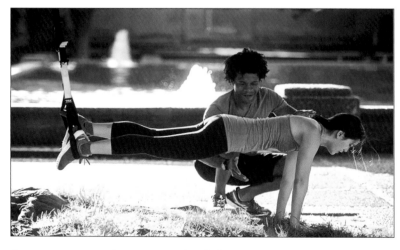

You see, when you incorporate unstable surfaces (medicine balls, suspension straps or the world itself), you must work extra hard in order to stabilize on your own. All the tiny muscles in the body must vibrate and harmonize a little bit extra for you to remain tense and solid.

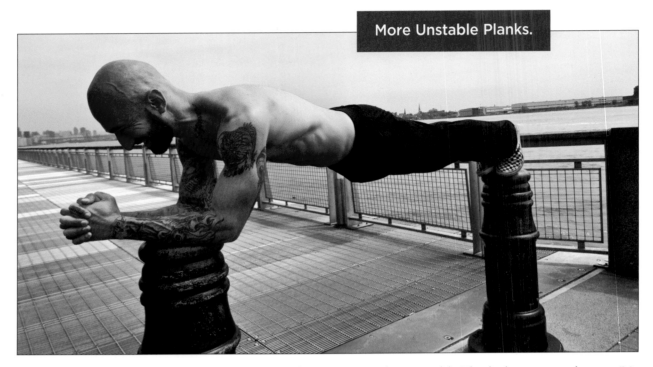

More Unstable Planks.

Trainer Talk: Generally, there is a lot more happening in the Unstable Plank than meets the eye. It's amazing how an exercise like this can make you break a sweat without any big movements.

Rep Range/Duration: Elite practitioners can hold isometric holds for seemingly indefinite amounts of time. I recommend getting to the point where Unstable Planks can be held for least 60 seconds.

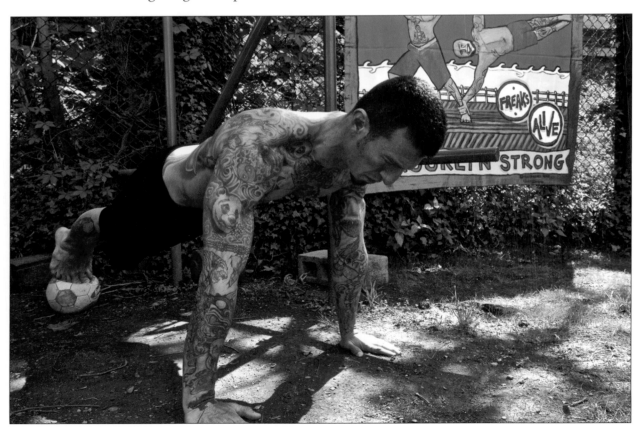

SEATED KNEE RAISE

The Seated Knee Raise a "missing link" of sorts between floor abs and hanging abs. Begin by sitting on the edge of a bench with your legs extended out in front of you. Use your abs to draw your knees in toward your chest. It is important that your upper body remain stable throughout the exercise. It may be helpful at the beginning to clasp the side of the bench with your hands.

Although some books list Seated Knee Raises as a "lower" abs exercise, I disagree. The whole body must truly work together to perform this exercise properly and with any degree of stability.

Trainer Talk: A popular variation involves twisting your knees to the side at the top of the motion, thus recruiting the obliques. Make sure to target both sides evenly.

Rep Range: 2 smooth, controlled sets of 20 is a solid stepping stone to hanging abs.

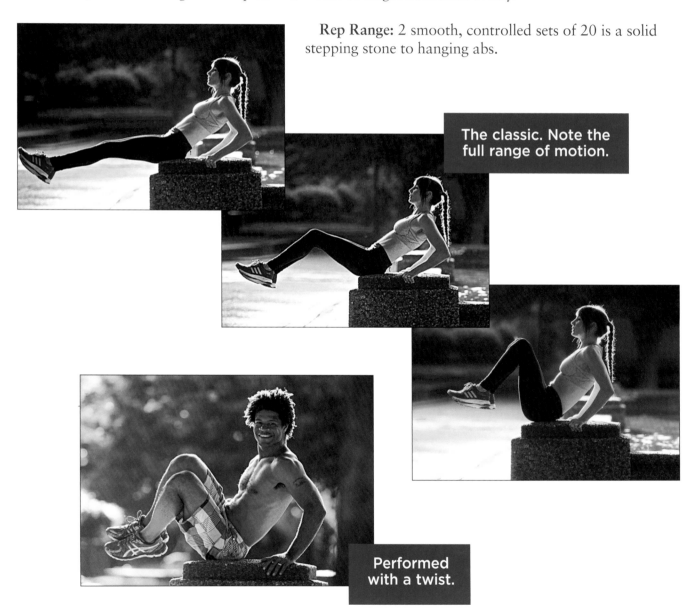

The classic. Note the full range of motion.

Performed with a twist.

N-SIT

Essentially, the N-Sit is an isometric hold at the top position of a Seated Knee Raise. In a seated position, raise your knees toward your chest. When they cannot come up any higher, find the balance and hold the top position. The N-Sit can be done just about anywhere. No gym is required.

Trainer Talk: The N-Sit can be thought of as a version of the L-Sit where the body is shortened, thus creating a slight mechanical advantage. The straighter you make your legs, the harder the exercise becomes.

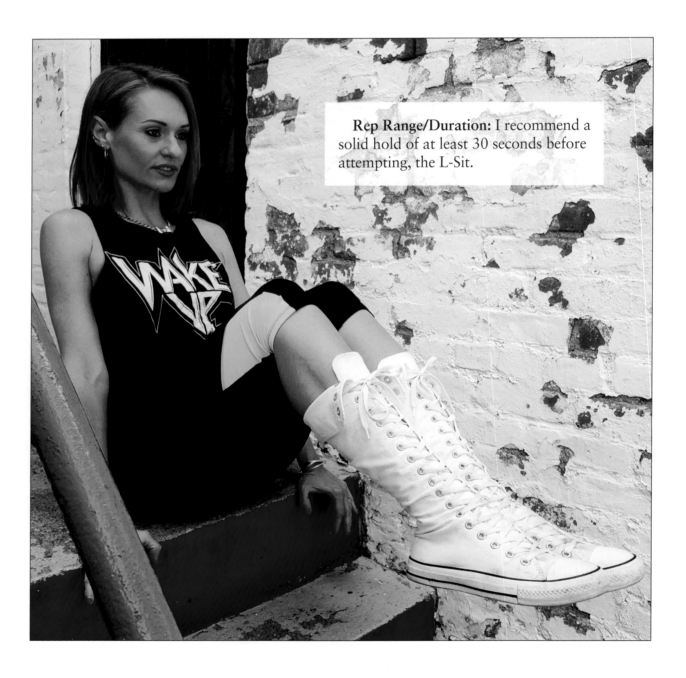

Rep Range/Duration: I recommend a solid hold of at least 30 seconds before attempting, the L-Sit.

GROUNDED WIPER

Fans of my work know that I adore classic Windshield Wipers. It's one of my all-time favorite bar calisthenic abs moves. However, it is a very ambitious exercise to jump right into. The Grounded Wiper allows you to rehearse the movement pattern on the floor before applying it to the bar. Think of it as a step between Lying Leg Raises and Hanging Windshield Wipers.

Begin by lying on the ground as with any Lying Leg Raise, then bring your legs to the top position, thighs perpendicular to the ground. I recommend keeping your hands (palms down) *wider* than you normally would in such a position. This will increase your "base". Now move both legs together from side to side. Left, center, right, center, continue. Keep it controlled. Work toward making that arc wide… Now you'll really feel that transverse twist!

If necessary, you can regress this exercise by flexing at the knees. The more the knees are bent, the shorter the body, hence, the easier the exercise. Conversely, this exercise is most challenging when performed with both legs completely straight. There are many variations in between.

Trainer Talk: Make sure to keep your shoulders and upper back flat on the floor for the entirety of the movement. Your left shoulder may want to come off the ground when you bring your feet to the right (and vice versa). Make a deliberate effort to maintain control.

Rep Range: Shoot for 10-20 reps, alternating sides.

THROWDOWN

Here's another old school classic. Because of the explosive effort unique to this exercise, Throwdowns are a part of many serious practitioners' arsenal.

With your partner standing above you, lie on the ground. Reach up and grab your partner's ankles. Tense up the body and raise your legs together, aggressively, toward your partner. The movement resembles that of a Lying Leg Raise, however, as your legs approach your partner, he puts his hands forth and "throws" your ankles back down to to the ground. Stop just short of touching the floor and repeat. You will feel this everywhere.

Trainer Talk: You can also perform Throwdowns with a twist to the right and left. The partner helps direct this movement. Make sure to communicate which variation you wish to perform, as with all partner assisted exercises.

Rep Range: When you can consistently do 3 sets of 15-20, give some of the early Advanced Abs exercises a try. Good luck!

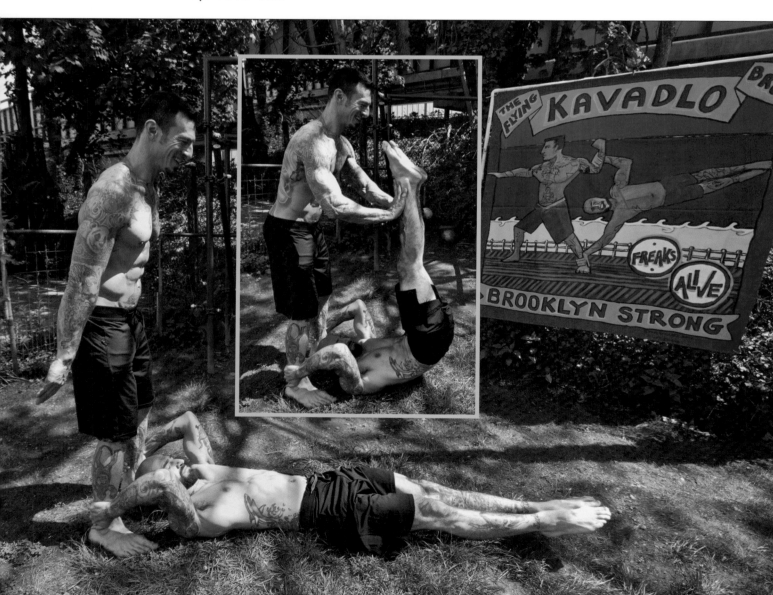

SIDE PLANK HIP RAISE

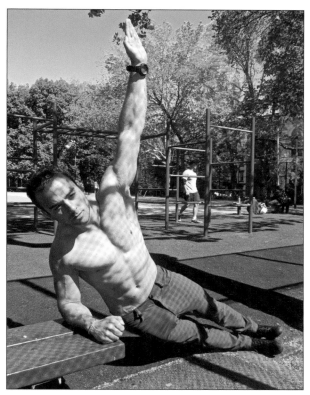

Make sure your standard Side Plank is solid before incorporating the hip raise. Now bring your hips high off the ground, vertically into the air as high as they will go. Lower them down slow and low. That is one rep. Make sure to train both sides evenly.

Side Plank Hip Raises are notorious for being deceptively challenging.

Trainer Talk: Like a standard Side Plank, you can incorporate a bench to adjust the leverage.

Rep Range: I recommend a solid 3 sets of 10 on each side before trying advanced exercises.

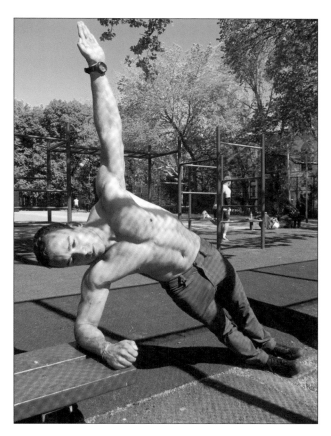

How to Hang

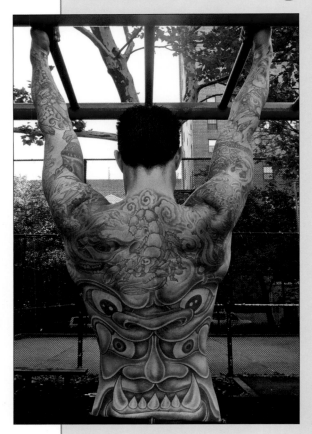

Grab the bar hard. This not only helps to initiate full body tension, it also establishes a strong, solid foundation. In fact, just actively hanging from the bar (sometimes called a "Bar Hang") can be considered an abs exercise in it's own right. When gripping the bar, it is important to keep your shoulder blades back and your chest up. Whether you choose an overhand, underhand or neutral grip, this tension and scapular retraction will help you get the most out of every single rep.

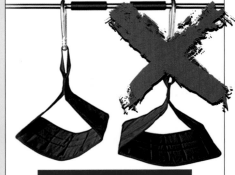

I am not a fan.

Some people will have a hard time hanging, particularly if they are overweight or new to working out. It is unlikely that these folks are ready for Advanced Abs in the first place. However, many choose to use Assistance Straps, and try anyway. I believe that it makes more sense to get better at floor abs, seated abs and simply hanging, than it does to use these whack straps. I generally do not like apparatuses that disconnect you from the surface on which you train, whether that surface is the bar, a bench or the world.

Almost all of the hanging abs exercises in this book can be done from a flex hang position. Essentially the top position of a pull-up, a flex hang can be executed from either a pronated (overhand), supinated (underhand) or combination (mixed) grip. Performing any of these abs exercises from a flex hang adds a unique neurological spin, and increases upper body muscle activation and energy expenditure. Highly recommended. Like the aforementioned active bar hang, simply getting into the Flex Hang position requires abdominal muscle recruitment.

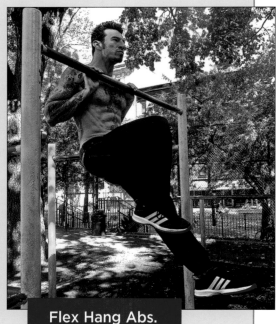

Flex Hang Abs.

Hanging Contest

The Hanging contest is exactly what it sounds like: a fun spin on the classic Bar Hang. Be mindful to keep and scapula retracted as you employ full body tension. Use every muscle in the body. Everyone's a winner in this contest.

Find a partner and a bar and let the fun begin!

Trainer Talk: The goal is to keep your body extended and your shoulders packed without twisting, turning or swinging. However, when hanging until muscular failure, it's natural for the form to deteriorate after an extended period of time.

Rep Range/Duration: As long as possible!

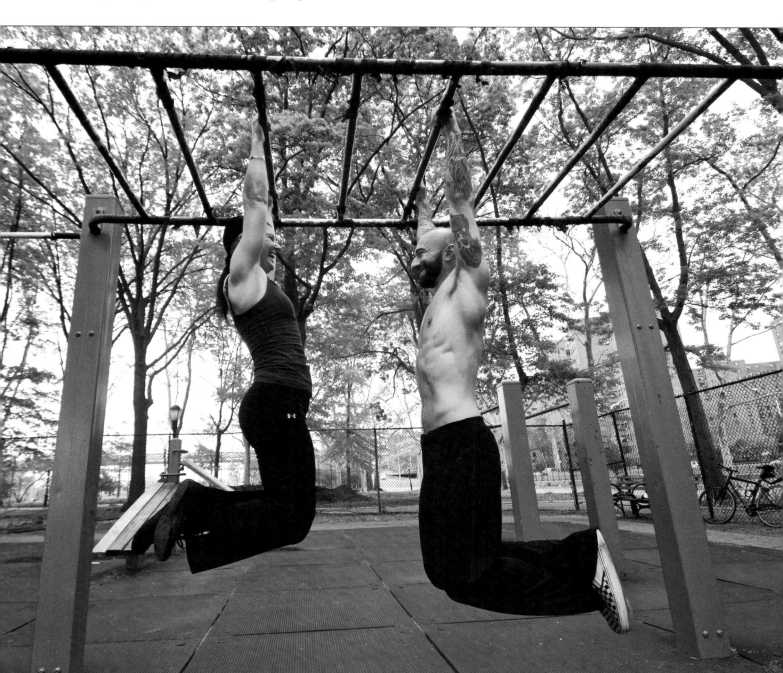

ONE ARM HANG

The One Arm Hang is virtually impossible to perform without a solid foundation of abdominal strength. Anyone who thinks it's not an abs exercise has never tried it. Start out by hanging from the bar with both arms. Keep your shoulders packed and every muscle in your body active. When you hang from the bar in this fashion, your entire body works together, with obvious emphasis on the arms. Now remove one hand from the bar and bring your arm to your side, all the while maintaining tension. The abs and glutes play a bigger role than one might assume. When you remove a hand from the equation, the abs must pick up a great deal of the slack.

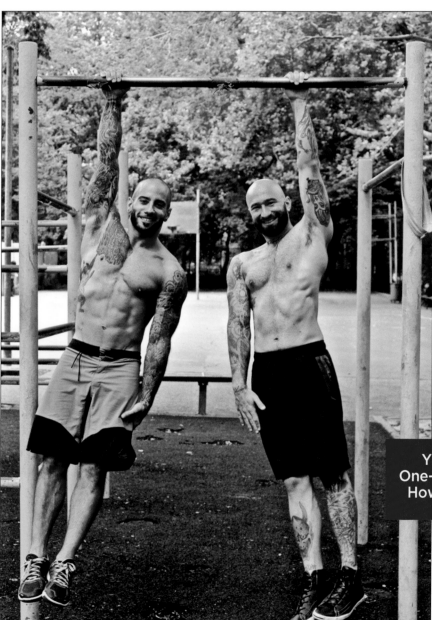

The goal is to keep your body extended and your shoulder packed without twisting, turning or swinging. Make sure to train both sides evenly.

Trainer Talk: In addition to your abs and glutes, activate your legs to avoid swinging from the lower body. Swinging can rob you of your energy. A strong grip is a prerequisite.

Rep Range/Duration: Upper body strength plays a huge role in how long one will be able to hang. Therefore, it varies greatly from individual to individual. It can be fun to hang for as long as you can.

> You can even have a
> One-Arm Hanging Contest.
> How long can you hang?

AB WHEEL ROLL-OUT (BENT KNEE)

An old time classic, Bent Knee Ab Wheel Roll-Outs incorporate stability, strength and focus in a truly unique way. They are also harder than they look. Start out in a kneeling position, holding the ab wheel apparatus in your hands. Place the wheel on the floor and pick up your hips, so that there is a straight line from your shoulder to your hip to your knee, which remains in contact with the ground. Roll the wheel out so that so that your arms move directly over your head and your torso lowers to the ground. It is crucial to maintain tension from the shoulders all the way down to the knees, not just in the abs, but in the entire core including the glutes, quads, back and chest. The farther you roll the wheel out, the more challenging this exercise becomes. When you have reached the bottom position, there will be about 6-8 inches between your chest and the ground, depending on the size of the wheel and your range of motion.

You can also roll the wheel out to the sides, veering toward the left or right, as opposed to straight overhead.

Trainer Talk: If you are new to this exercise then you may need to start with only a partial range of motion. That is okay, as long as the goal of full range of motion is met before attempting the more advanced Straight Leg Ab Wheel Roll-Outs.

Rep Range: It is a good idea to perform 2-4 sets of 10 reps. Listen to your body; this can take longer to achieve than it may seem.

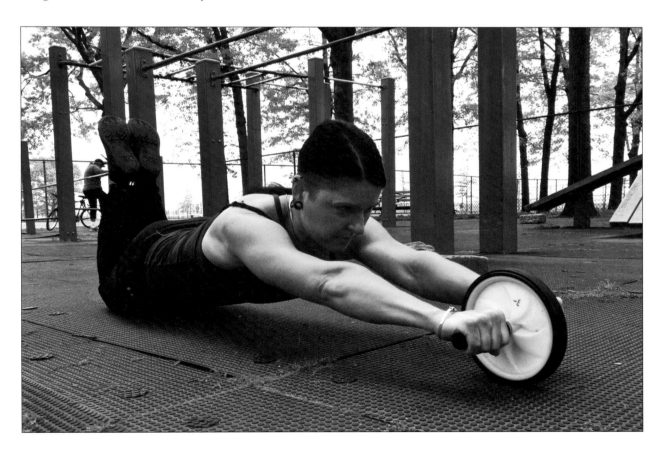

HANGING BICYCLE

For many people, the elusive Hanging Bicycle is the last progression before achieving the Hanging Knee Raise, considered to be the standard of basic abdominal calisthenic prowess.

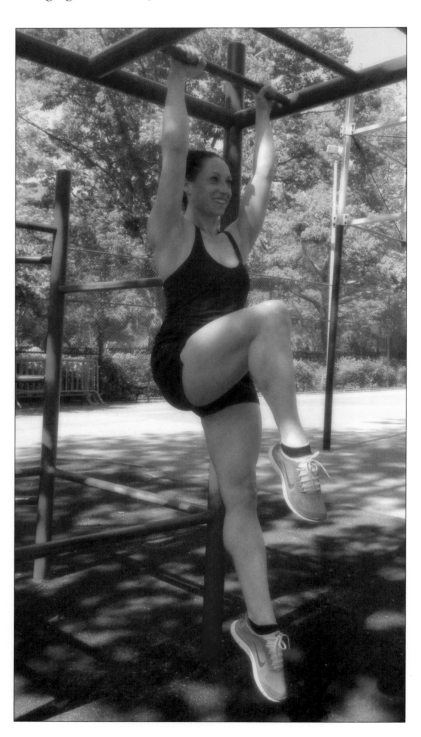

Start by hanging from the bar. Raise your knees alternately past waist height one at a time. The transition should be smooth, like the motion of pedaling a real bicycle. Like Lying Bicycles, this exercise is a more forgiving than keeping both feet together.

Trainer Talk: Common mistakes include "pedaling" too quickly. The extra force generated by the speed may become your enemy. One of the keys to bar abs excellence is the ability to control momentum… instead of it controlling you!

Rep Range/Duration: A good short term goal is 30-40 (15-20 per side) reps. Because reps go by quickly, I sometimes I like to challenge myself by "pedaling" for time instead of reps. Aim for 30 seconds, then one minute, etc. Push the limits.

HANGING KNEE RAISE

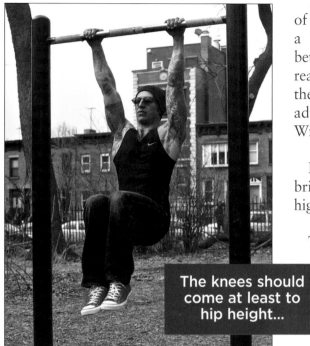

The Hanging Knee Raise is one of the most important of all abdominal exercises. It is considered by many to be a "gatekeeper" of sorts, a proverbial stepping stone between *intermediate* and *advanced*. It is only after a reaching a certain level of comfort and confidence with the Hanging Knee Raise that one should even consider advanced moves like Straight Leg Raises, Front Levers, Windshield Wipers or Dragon Flags.

Begin by hanging from the bar. In a controlled fashion, bring both knees up together. Your knees should come up higher than your hip. Aim for the chest.

Trainer Talk: This exercise has more subtlety to it than one might think. It can be helpful to point your toes slightly in front of you at the bottom range of motion, rather than straight down. This will help you control momentum, particularly on the first few reps, which can make you or break you.

The knees should come at least to hip height...

Rep Range: 20 consecutive reps is a considered to be a solid baseline.

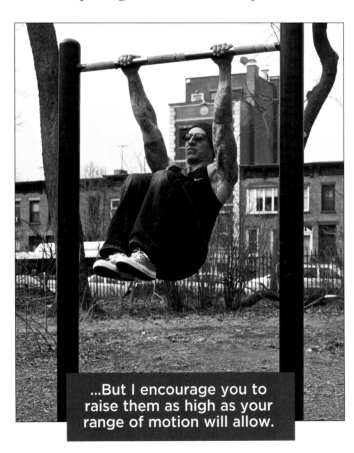

...But I encourage you to raise them as high as your range of motion will allow.

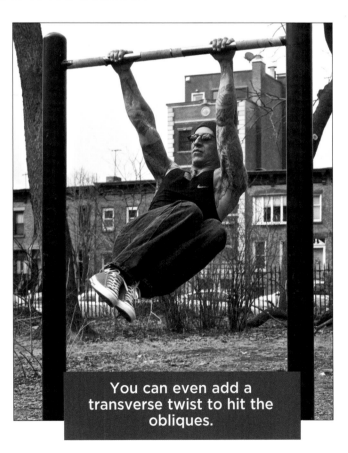

You can even add a transverse twist to hit the obliques.

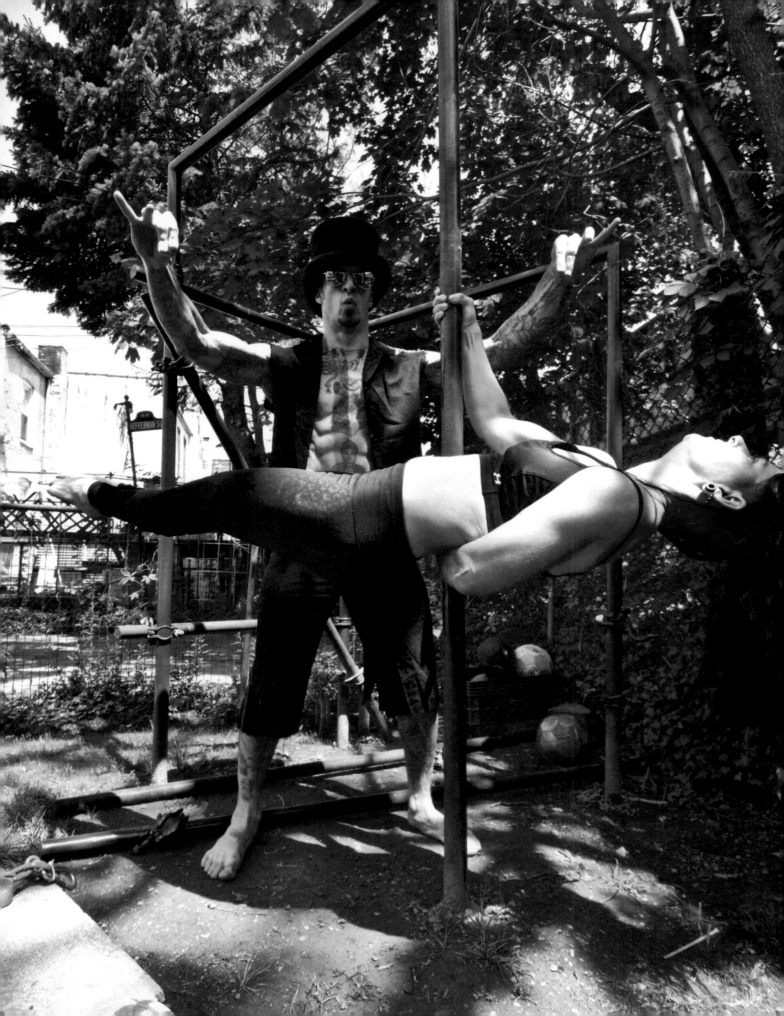

ADVANCED ABS

Here's some *serious* stuff. Moving forward, you will no longer find the terms "upper" or "lower" at all. These moves are all full body, baby. Emphasis everywhere. Although the following exercises put tremendous demand on the abs, you will find the need for complete strength and harmony all over, no division between mind and muscle.

You may also require more recovery time even if you are performing fewer reps. That's okay; five Dragon Flags trumps fifty Lying Single Leg Raises.

L-SIT

The L-Sit has its origins in gymnastics but has been widely adapted by the calisthenics and Street Workout community. Sometimes you even see it in the big box gyms. With your hands on the floor and in a seated position, press down into the ground with your legs extended directly out in front of you.

As you contract from your abs, your pelvis will tilt forward and your hips will shift in front of you. You will feel this exercise everywhere.

L-Sits can also be performed on parallel bars, pull-up bars, kettlebells or just about any object. Each one has its own characteristics.

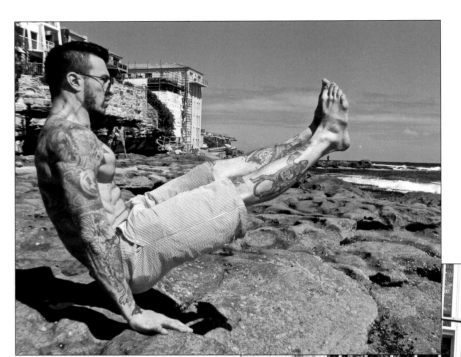

Trainer Talk: To obtain the greatest mechanical advantage, rotate your elbow pits, or "eyes of the elbows" out in front of you, rather than inwardly and keep your arms close to your torso.

Rep Range/Duration: 30 seconds is respectable. One minute is advanced.

L-Sits can be done on many surfaces, to varying degrees.

GECKO HOLD

It may be helpful to think of the Gecko Hold as a "limited contact" Plank. Typical Gecko Holds involve the use of only one arm and one leg as points of contact, thus creating a stability challenge on the muscles that cross your trunk. This 1-arm, 1-leg position is said to resemble the movement of the elusive desert gecko, wily in its ways.

A ripped six-pack is nothing without strength. Gecko Holds place a unique challenge on the trainee.

Trainer Talk: The Gecko Hold takes some getting used to. Some people find it helpful to keep both feet together until they are comfortable taking one foot off the ground. Gecko Holds can further be modified by using your forearm as a point of contact, rather than your hand. This provides more stability, but less favorable leverage.

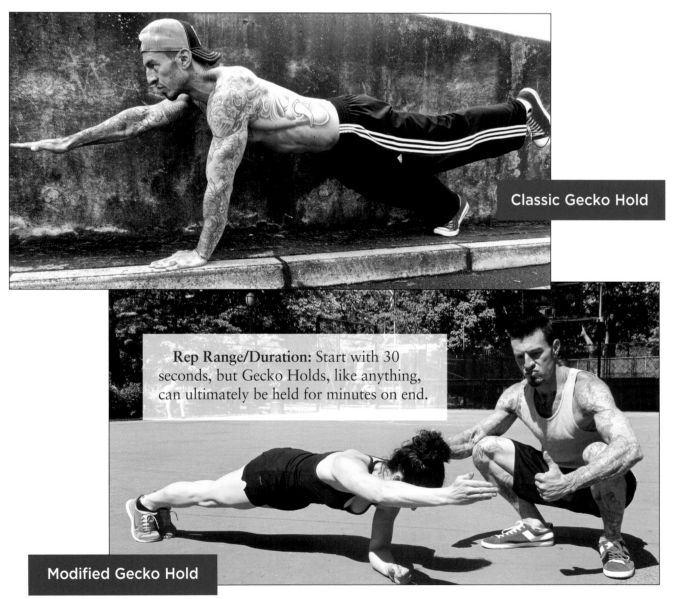

Classic Gecko Hold

Rep Range/Duration: Start with 30 seconds, but Gecko Holds, like anything, can ultimately be held for minutes on end.

Modified Gecko Hold

AB WHEEL ROLL-OUT (STRAIGHT LEG)

These are just like the bent knee variety, only much more difficult. Hold the ab wheel in front of you and, from a standing position, lower it to the ground. Allow your arms to go over your head as the wheel rolls out in front of you. Keep your legs straight the whole time. The farther you roll the wheel out, the more challenging this exercise becomes. When your arms are overhead and you hips are close to the ground, return to the starting position by bringing the wheel back in and "piking" your hips into the air.

This exercise is incredibly challenging for practitioners of all fitness levels. Full body tension is key.

Trainer Talk: If you are new to this exercise then you may need to start with only a partial range of motion. It may be a long time before full range of motion is achieved. This exercise can also be regressed by spreading your feet apart into a "straddle" position. This shortens the length of the body creating more favorable leverage.

Rep Range: A good goal is 2-4 sets of 5. Listen to your body; this may take longer to achieve than it may seem. For many, 1-2 clean reps will prove to be extremely challenging.

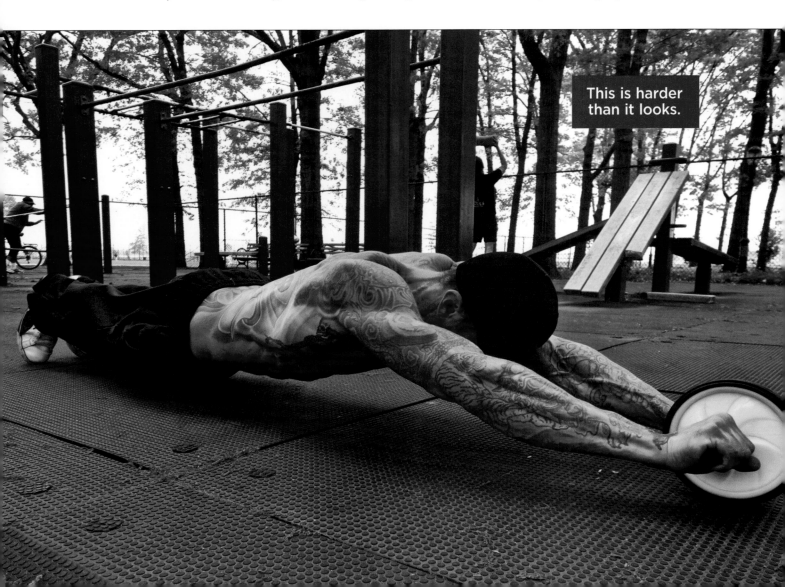

This is harder than it looks.

HANGING LEG RAISE

This is one of my all-time favorites. Here's where we take the Hanging Knee Raise to the next level. Start by hanging from the bar. While maintaining straight legs, use your abs to bring your legs all the way up until your shins come into contact with the bar. Lower them back down and repeat. (A regressed version involves bringing the legs up until they are parallel to the ground.) Both versions are an excellent pre-cursor to Windshield Wipers.

Obviously, this exercise requires more than just abdominal power; you will also need to engage the arms and back (particularly the lats and long head of the triceps) to help facilitate the full range of motion.

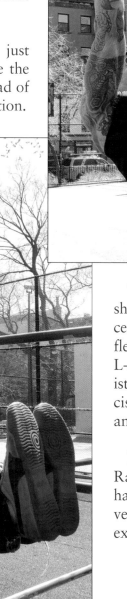

...or all the way to the bar!

You can bring your legs parallel to the ground...

Trainer Talk: To get your shins all the way to the bar, a certain degree of hamstring flexibility is required. Like the L-Sit (and much advanced calisthenics in general), this exercise requires both strength and mobility.

Rep Range: Hanging Leg Raises can be deceptively hard. Six controlled reps is very good. Ten or more is excellent.

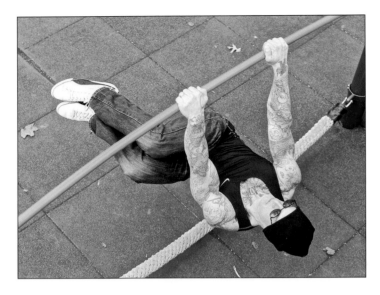

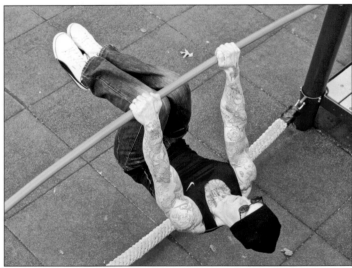

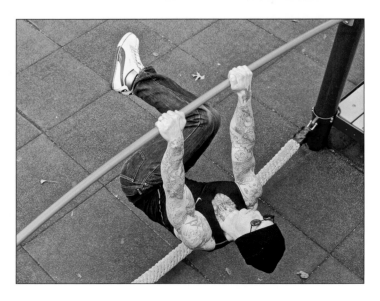

WASHING MACHINE

The infamous Washing Machine is more advanced than the Hanging Knee Raise with a Twist. It's widely regarded as a key stepping stone toward the mighty Windshield Wiper, as they are similar movement patterns. The Washing Machine simply incorporates flexion at the knees and hips, thus shortening the body and allowing for more forgiving leverage.

Hang from the bar and bring your knees up so they're at hip height. With your legs squeezed together, rotate the knees to the left, then back to the middle and towards the right. Do not return to a straight leg position until the completion of the set.

Trainer Talk: Sometimes referred to as "The Spin Cycle", this exercise can be regressed by bringing your knees high up toward the chest, rather than shins parallel to the ground. This creates a smaller angle at the hip and knee, thus shortening length of the body.

Rep Range: When you feel comfortable with ten to twenty reps, it's Windshield Wiper time.

WINDSHIELD WIPER

The first time someone attempts Windshield Wipers, they are often unprepared for how much upper body strength is required. Brace yourself!

Start out in the top position of a Hanging Leg Raise. While squeezing the bar tightly and keeping your legs (and knees) together, rotate your straight legs to the left, then back to the center and toward the right.

Increase the difficulty by increasing the range of motion. In other words, bringing your feet out farther from your body will force you to work harder. Take your time with Windshield Wipers. Even for advanced fitness practitioners, Windshield Wiper mastery takes a long time.

Trainer Talk: Controlling your own body weight is important here; squeeze the bar hard! You may also notice a slight bend in the elbow on the side that you are rotating toward. Try to keep your arms as straight as possible to keep the emphasis on the abs, but slight kinking of the elbow is often unavoidable.

Rep Range: Start out with sets of 2-4 reps at a time. 3 sets of 10 is a solid goal. 3 sets of 20 is advanced.

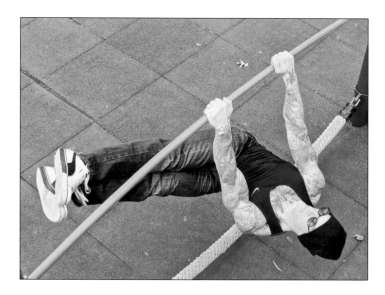

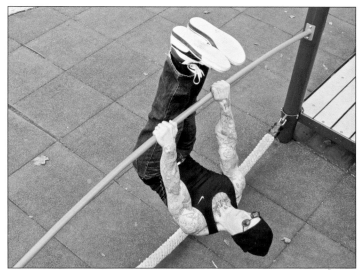

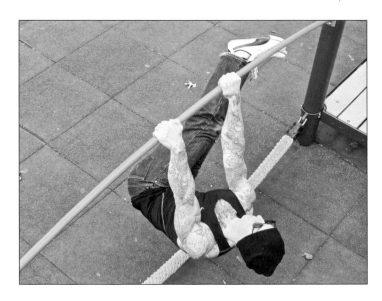

V-LEG WIPER

This exercise is very similar to the classic Windshield Wiper. The key distinction is that the legs are kept apart, in a "V" formation. Since there will be less overall tension (from not squeezing your legs together), the core must compensate.

Trainer Talk: Prepare to feel more emphasis in the glutes than you may expect. It is necessary to stabilize.

Rep Range: Like the classic Windshield Wiper, 3 sets of 10-20 reps are good goals, but you will have to start with 2-4 at a time.

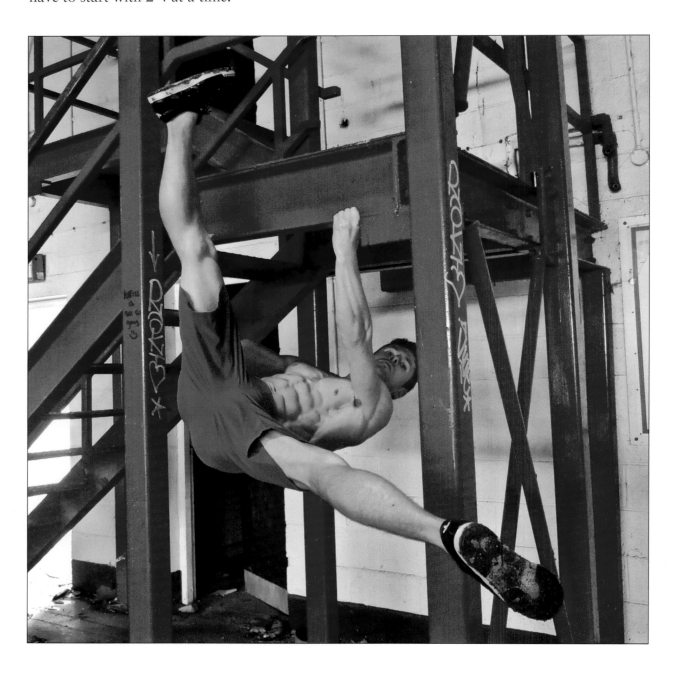

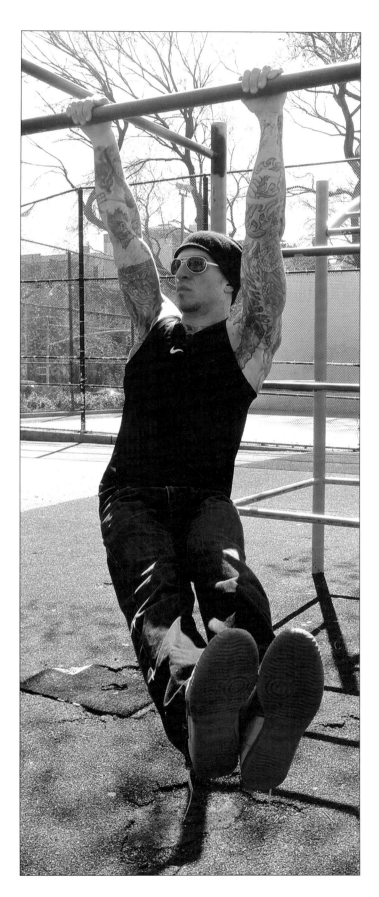

PERFECT CIRCLE

Ultimately, this is an exaggerated Windshield Wiper. Instead of moving your legs side to side like the windshield wiper of an automobile, move your legs around your entire body forming a complete, giant circle with your feet. Pause every 360 degrees when your feet are straight up in the top position. Now rotate the other direction.

Trainer Talk: Make sure to keep the legs together at the knees, not just the feet. Squeeze the bar hard to initiate full body tension.

Rep Range: 3 sets of 10 (5 reps in each direction) is very solid.

SKINNING THE CAT

Skinning The Cat is a pre-cursor to many extreme bar calisthenics moves and a phenomenal abs exercise in its own right. Start off by hanging from the bar. Slowly begin to lift your knees as you would in a Hanging Knee Raise. However, continue to bring your knees up until they pass your chest. Follow through with the motion until you can pull them toward the bar and ultimately under and past it. After your feet are on the other side of the bar, continue the motion until your toes are pointing to the ground. Now reverse the entire process. The reversal may prove more difficult than the initiation.

In gymnastics, this exercise must be performed with a supinated (underhand) grip. As a practitioner of Street Workout with no formal gymnastics training, either grip is okay with me. If you do choose to use a traditional gymnast grip, be prepared for additional tension on the biceps tendon. Further concerning grip, be careful not to grab the bar too wide. A narrower grip will allow you more space to get your legs under and past the bar.

Trainer Talk: If you are new to this exercise, you may experience difficulty bringing your feet all the way under the bar smoothly, even with a narrow grip. If this is the case, you might need to "kick through", using your feet to push you're your hips under and to the other side of the bar. That's okay. This will improve over time.

Rep Range: I enjoy doing five or six solid, slow reps at a time, but feel free to do more if you wish. More than ten at a time may be unnecessary. The bottom position, sometimes called a "German Hang" makes a great stretch for shoulders and upper back.

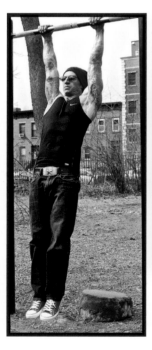 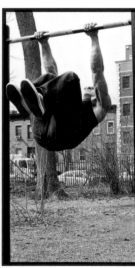 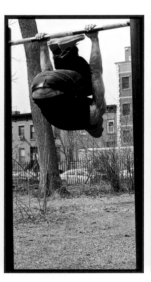 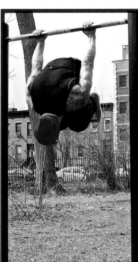 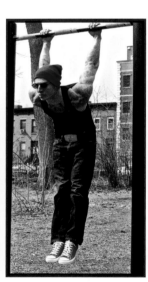

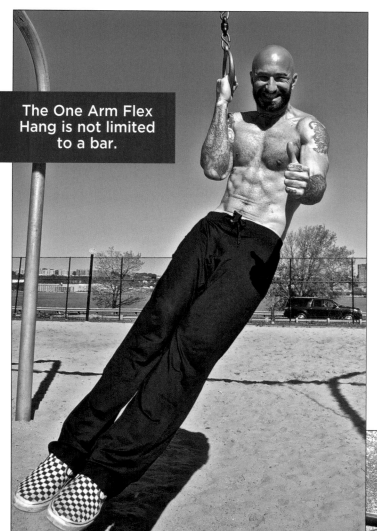

The One Arm Flex Hang is not limited to a bar.

ONE ARM FLEX HANG

Clearly, anyone who performs a One Arm Flex Hang has an incredibly strong upper body. But even more so, its practitioners must possess an inherent degree of muscular control and neurological communication. As we mentioned at the end of Chapter 17, the standard Flex Hang (using both arms) is an abs exercise in itself.

Start out at the top Pull-Up, in the standard Flex Hang position. Brace your abs, right arm and entire body as you prepare to remove your left hand. When you remove the hand, actively pull the bar toward you, squeezing with your entire body. Make sure to practice it on both sides.

This exercise is incredibly challenging. Full body tension and a strong grip are necessary.

Trainer Talk: Even when actively pulling the bar toward your body, be prepared to fall from the top position quickly if you are new to this exercise. It may be helpful to think of it as a slow negative One Arm Pull-Up. Respect the move and take your time.

Rep Range/Duration: At the beginning, a hold of any duration is good. 10-20 seconds or more is excellent.

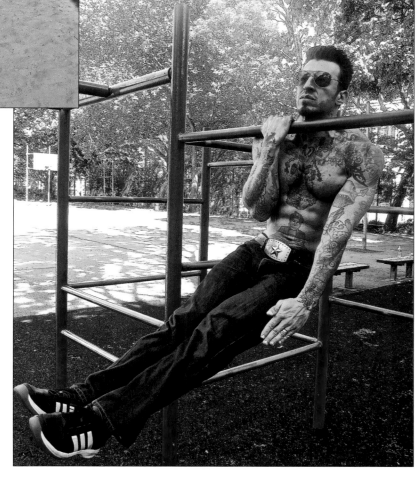

DRAGON FLAG

The Dragon Flag is an advanced calisthenics staple, a killer core exercise and a spectacular visual! Start by laying back on a bench. Reach up and overhead, grabbing the end of the bench with your hands. This will keep you from tipping over. Now, keep your body straight and unflexed at the hip and raise your body into the air. Unlike a Lying Leg Raise, the fulcrum point of the Dragon Flag is at the shoulder blades, not the hip.

Trainer Talk: The Dragon Flag can also be performed without a bench, as long as there is something for the practitioner to hold onto, be it a pole, partner or random object.

Rep Range: I prefer the Dragon Flag as an isometric exercise. A 5-10 second hold is a great place to start, with 30 seconds being a solid goal. But the Dragon Flag can also be done for reps. I recommend 4-10 as a goal, but just start with one and try to make it nice.

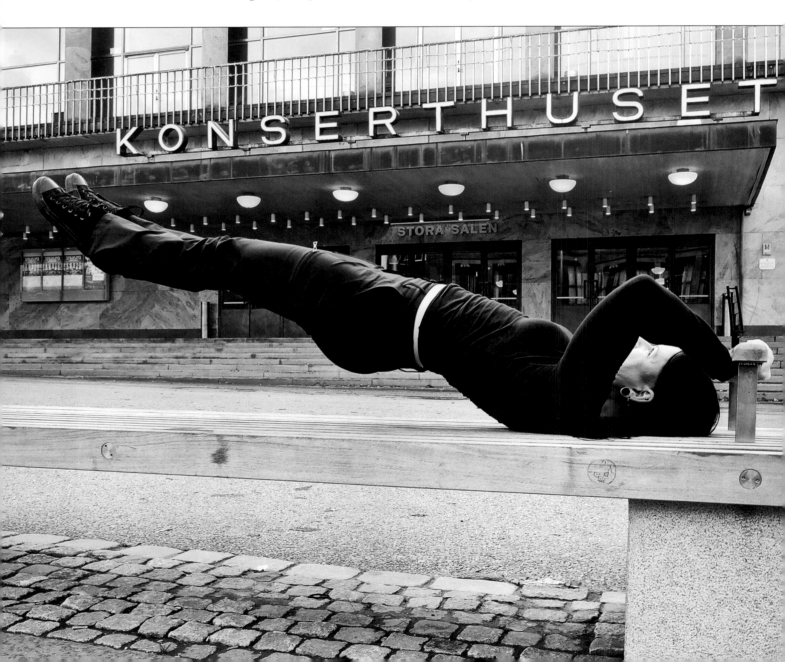

TUCK FRONT LEVER

All bar levers are elite calisthenics moves. The Tuck Front Lever is no exception. Along with its variations, the Tuck Front Lever can ultimately be progressed to the full Front Lever, where you keep your entire body straight and parallel to the ground, face up, with your hands on the bar. It can take months or even years to achieve.

The Tuck Front Lever is a regressed version where both your knees are tucked up toward the chest. Shoulders and hips are still parallel to the ground, as with the full Front Lever. Start out hanging from the bar, with your knees up, like the top position of a Hanging Knee Raise. Bring your knees up while simultaneously, and with straight arms, pull the bar down to your waist. Your upper body should be parallel to the ground.

In addition to abdominal strength, bar levers require a brutal level of upper body power.

Trainer Talk: There are varying degrees of tuck. The farther your knees are tucked toward your upper body, the more the exercise is regressed. Conversely, greater leg extension intensifies the exercise. You can even try one leg tucked or bicycle tucks, as "hidden steps" toward the Front Lever.

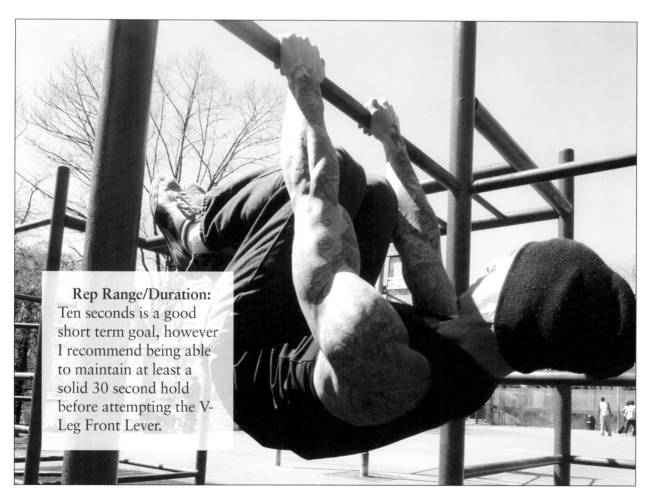

Rep Range/Duration: Ten seconds is a good short term goal, however I recommend being able to maintain at least a solid 30 second hold before attempting the V-Leg Front Lever.

V-LEG FRONT LEVER

Keeping your legs apart in a "V" or "straddle" formation is another way of shortening the body. As with the Tuck Front Lever, this will provide more favorable leverage than keeping them out in front of you, as you would in a full Front Lever. Start by hanging from the bar. Now, with straight arms, pull the bar down toward your waist as you spread your legs apart. Ultimately our upper body should be parallel to the ground, with your feet in a wide stance.

Trainer Talk: When you begin feeling comfortable in a wide straddle, try bringing your feet in closer together. You are on your way.

Rep Range/Duration: This is an extremely difficult move. Initially, just a few seconds will be challenging. Ten seconds or longer is excellent.

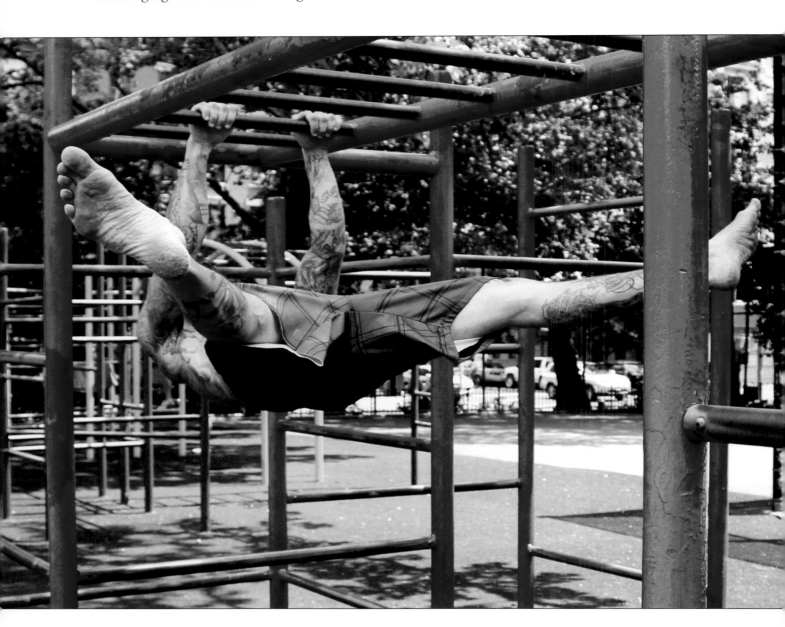

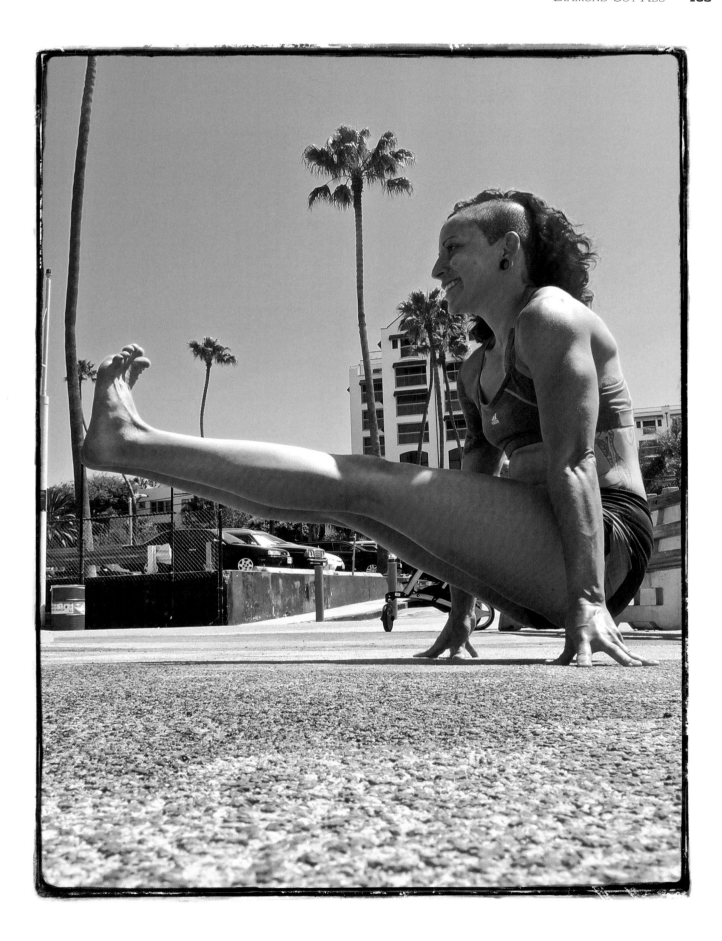

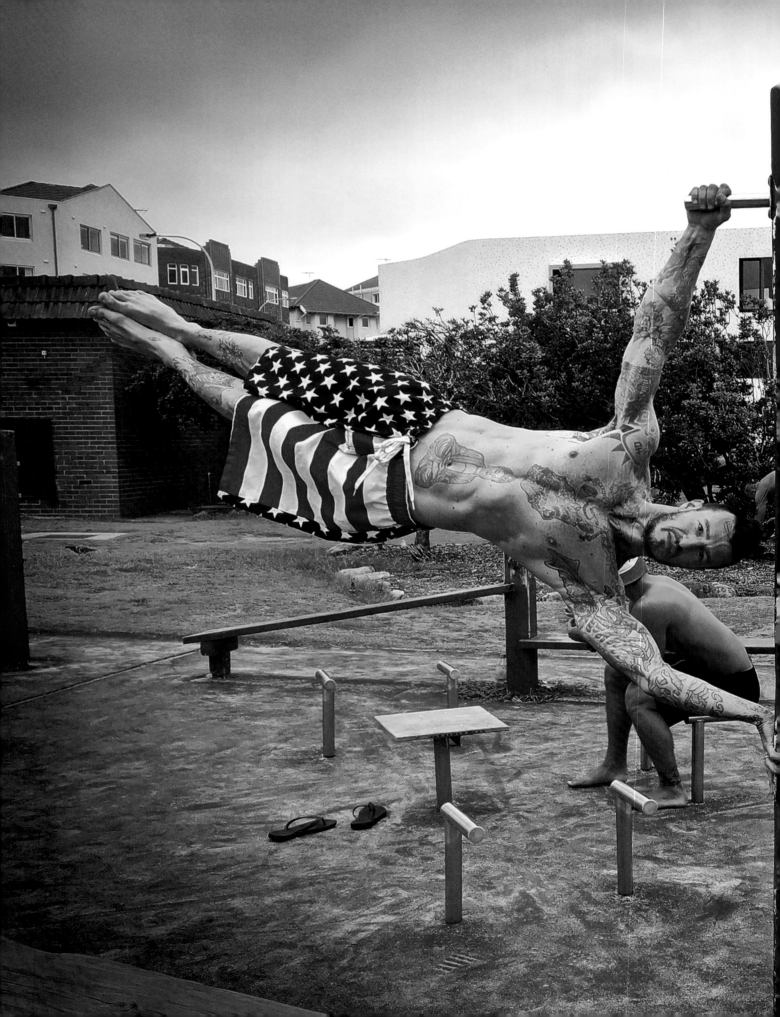

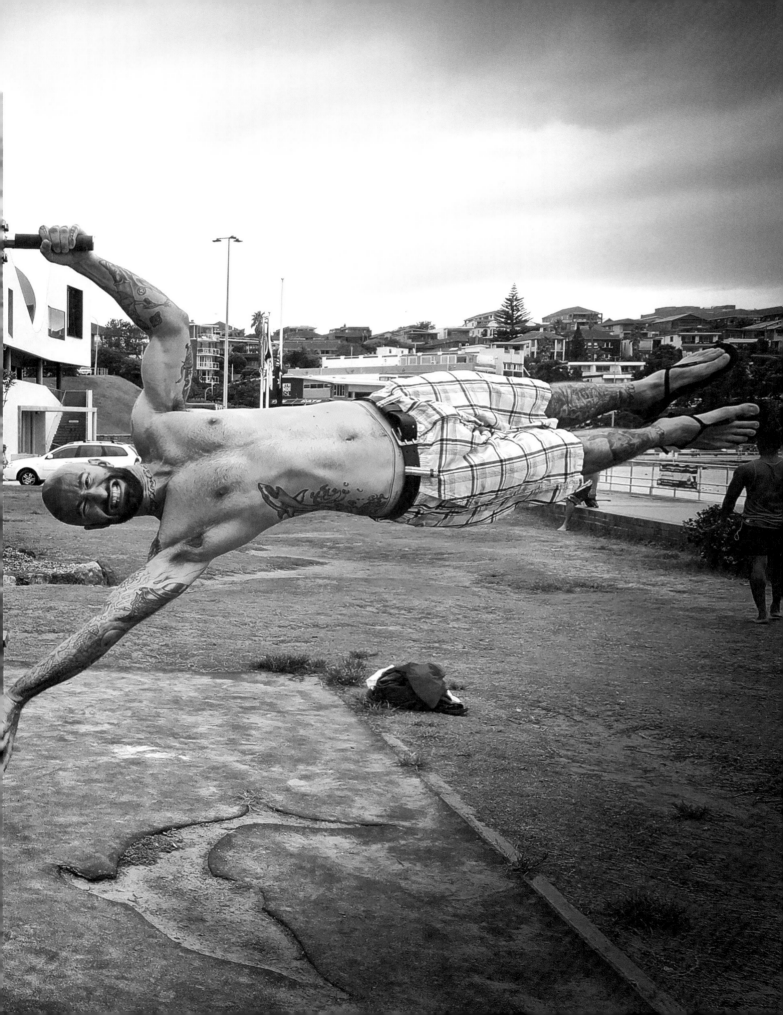

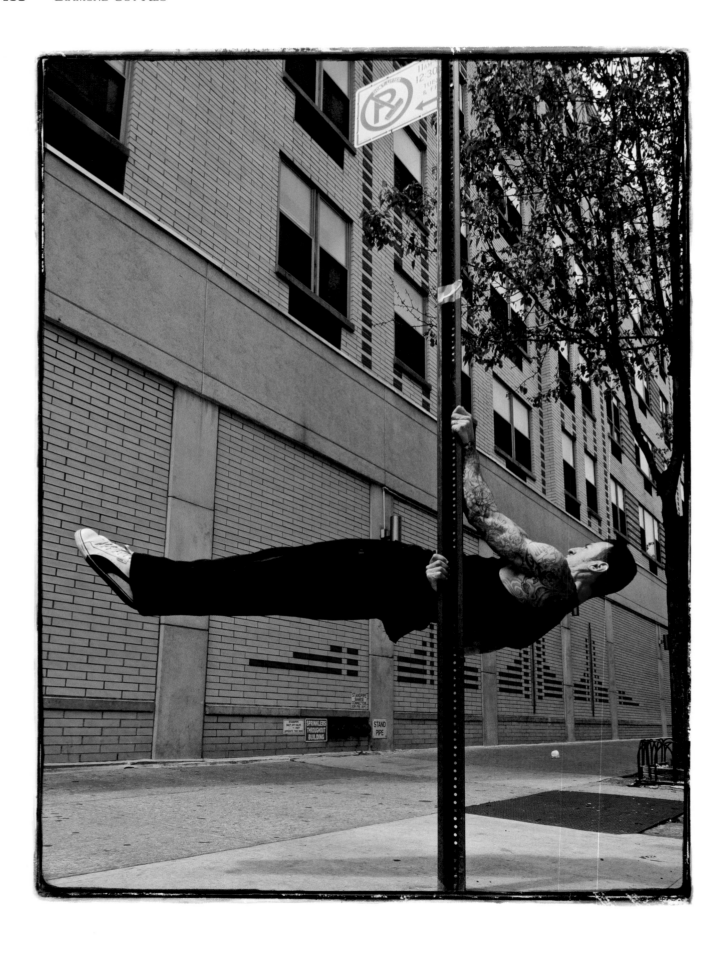

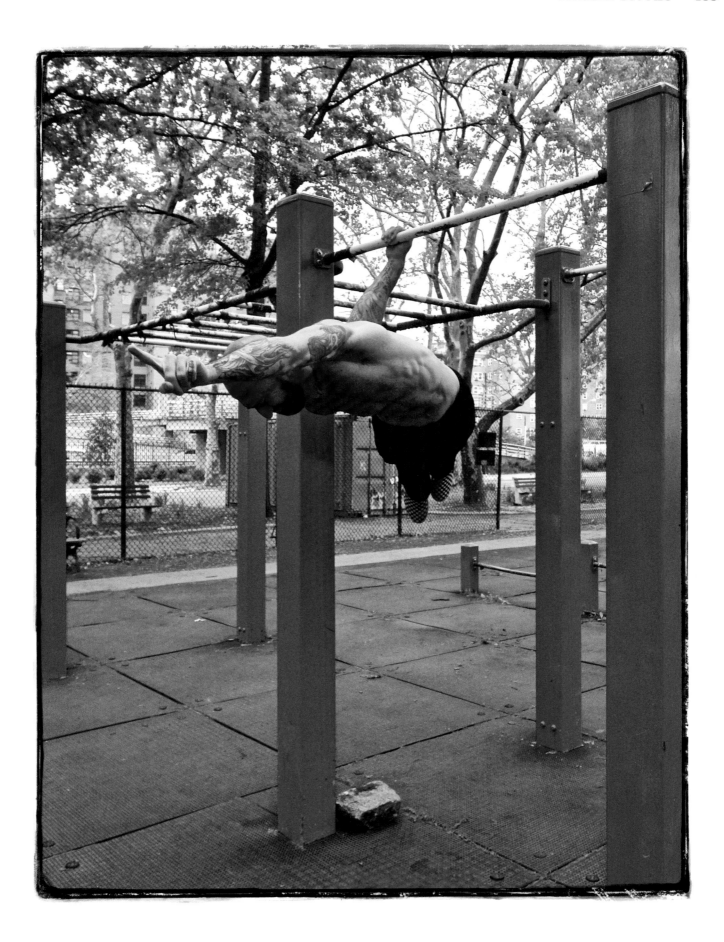

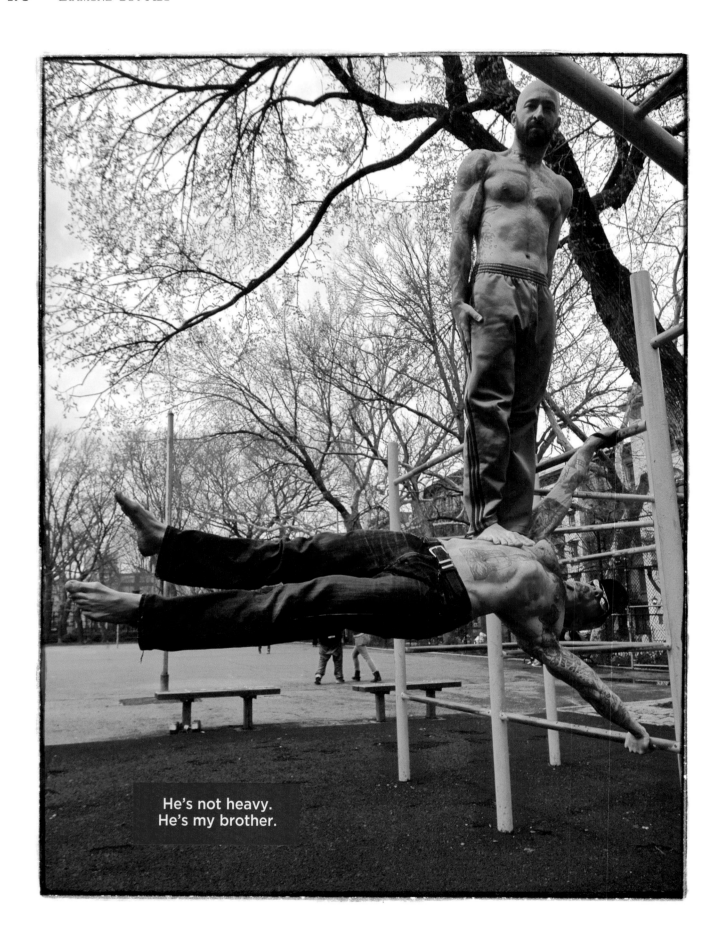

He's not heavy.
He's my brother.

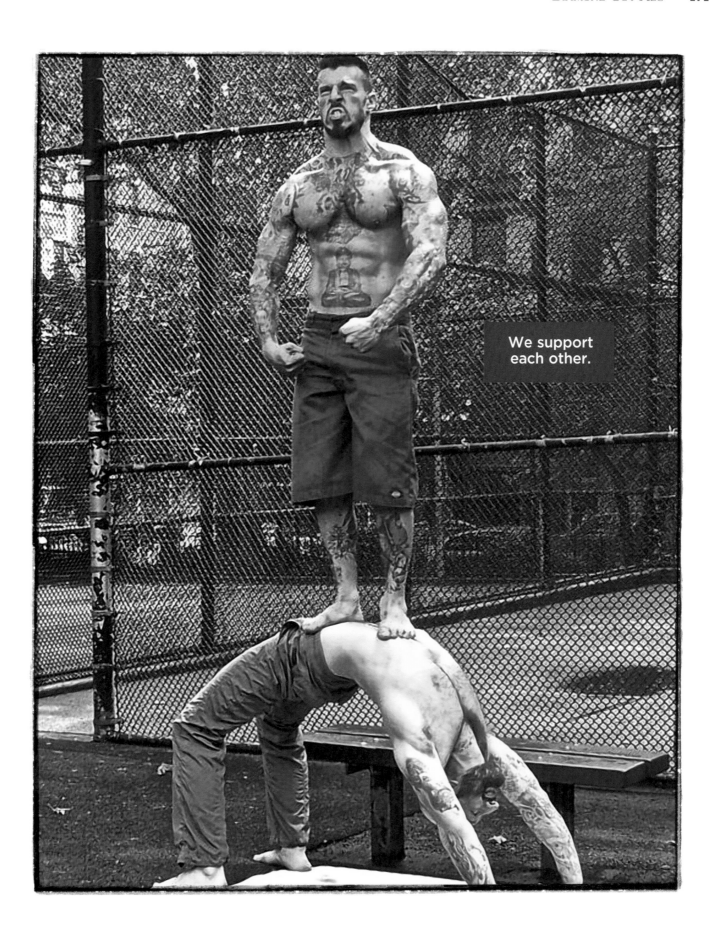

We support
each other.

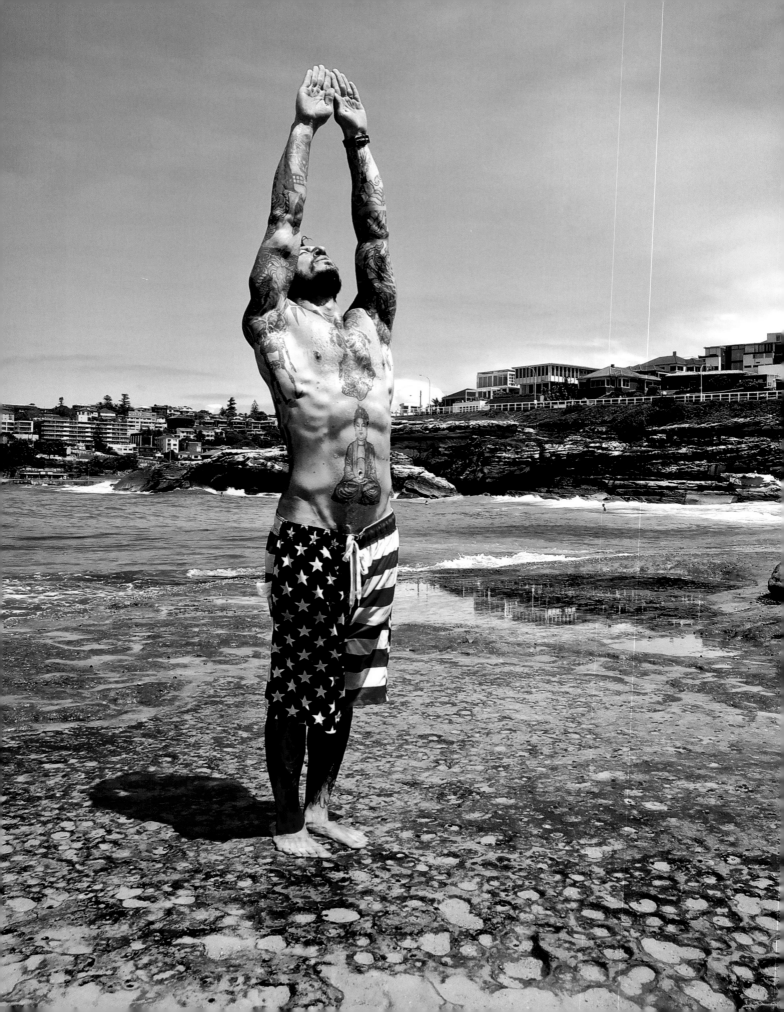

SUPPLEMENTAL STRETCHES

Stretching is very important. It helps open your joints and administer blood to your muscles and connective tissue. It helps enable your range of motion. I find that stretching before a workout prepares my mind/body connection for the training about to ensue. It even gets me ready emotionally.

Stretching after a workout has numerous benefits too. It allows your muscles, tendons and ligaments to cool down, as well as providing an "opposite reaction" to strength training. This helps facilitate quicker gains, improves recovery time and promotes mobility.

These stretches can be done before, during and/or after your workout. They should be held for several deep breaths at a time.

HANDS UP

This is usually how I begin my workouts. Not only does this one stretch out your abs, but almost every other muscle in your body as well. It's also excellent for increasing shoulder mobility, which will help all hanging abs training (and life in general).

Start out by standing in a narrow stance. Press your feet into the ground and lift your hands overhead, with arms extended. Keep your chest up, and look to the sky. Reach up and stretch deep. Breathe several deep breaths.

Trainer Talk: Some folks prefer to clasp their hands together at the top in order to facilitate a deeper stretch in the shoulders. Find what works best for you.

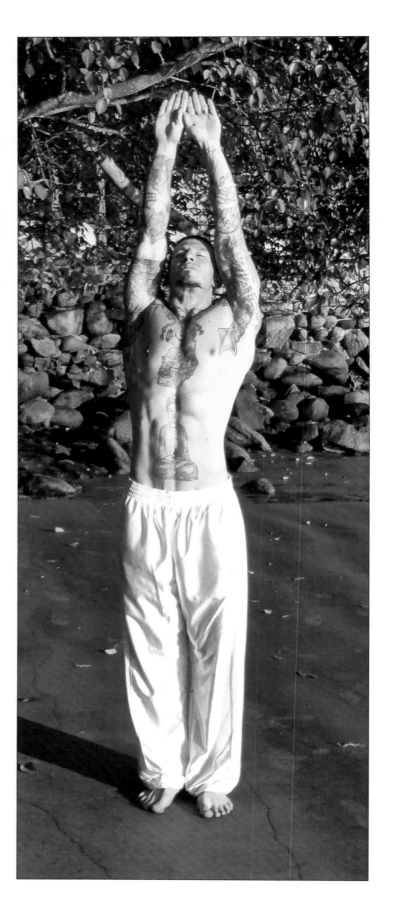

FORWARD, BACK & SIDE-TO-SIDE BEND

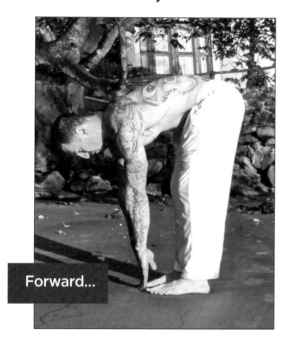

Forward...

Start at the top of the Hands Up stretch. Now bend forward, allowing your back to decompress as we stretch entire posterior chain of the body. Take your time. It feels good. Next, lean back in the opposite direction. Reach behind you with your chest up, pushing your hips in front of you. You'll feel this all the way through your abs and entire front of your body. Finally, reach your arms to the left, bending your whole body. Feel the deep stretch. Now move back to the center and reach your arms to the right. This side-to-side stretch is great after Crossovers, Windshield Wipers and anything that targets the obliques. Do this as many times as necessary.

Trainer Talk: Try not shrug your shoulders or bend too much at your knees when bending forward, although some beginners may have to bend a little if their hamstrings are inflexible.

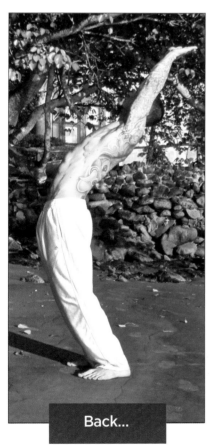

Back...

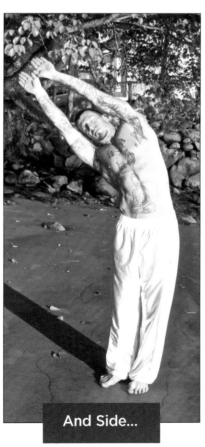

And Side...

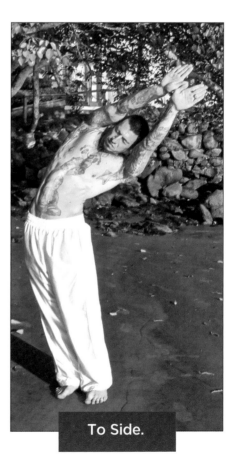

To Side.

HANDS DOWN

This is another fantastic stretch for the entire front of the body, particularly the abs. I enjoy holding this pose and breathing deeply.

From the top of a Push-Up position, lower your hips to the ground. Depending on your degree of spinal mobility, you may have to bend your arms at the elbows; this is fine, as long as they're not flaring out to the sides. (You can even do this stretch completely bent at the elbow, with your forearms on the ground if that's what is appropriate.) Now pull your chest forward and up, keeping your shoulder blades back and down. Actively press down with your hands, as the name implies, while keeping your hips close to the ground.

Trainer Talk: This stretch can potentially put some compression on the lumbar spine. Be mindful. Supplement this stretch with Forward Bends.

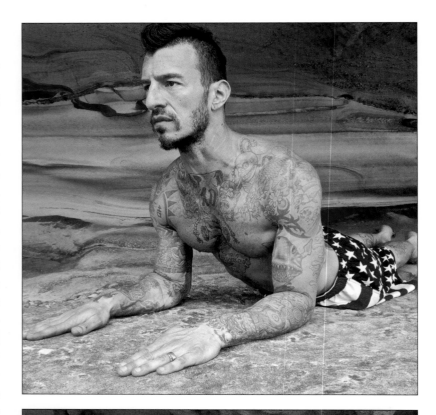

Depending on spinal flexibility, this stretch can be performed with arms fully extended, bent to 90 degrees, or anywhere in between.

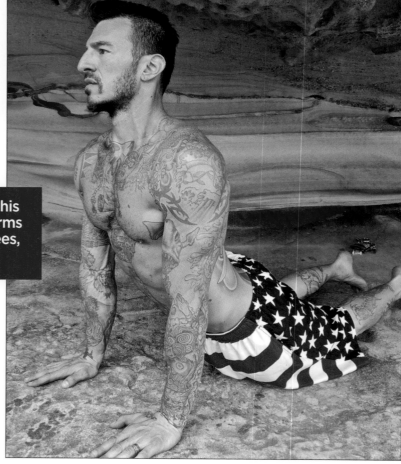

SEATED TWIST

The Seated Twist targets the abs and lower back—not to mention shoulders, hips and chest. First sit down with your legs out in front of you. Bend your left knee and cross your left leg over your right. Reach over with your right arm and put it against your left knee, pushing your chest out to your left. Turn your head toward the left shoulder as you rotate your trunk in the same direction. Keep your back straight and your chest high. Hold this for several breaths. Repeat on the right side. It's important to stretch each side evenly.

Trainer Talk: Make sure you have your left hand and foot pressed flat on the ground when twisting to the left. Apply the same practice to your right hand and foot when twisting to the right.

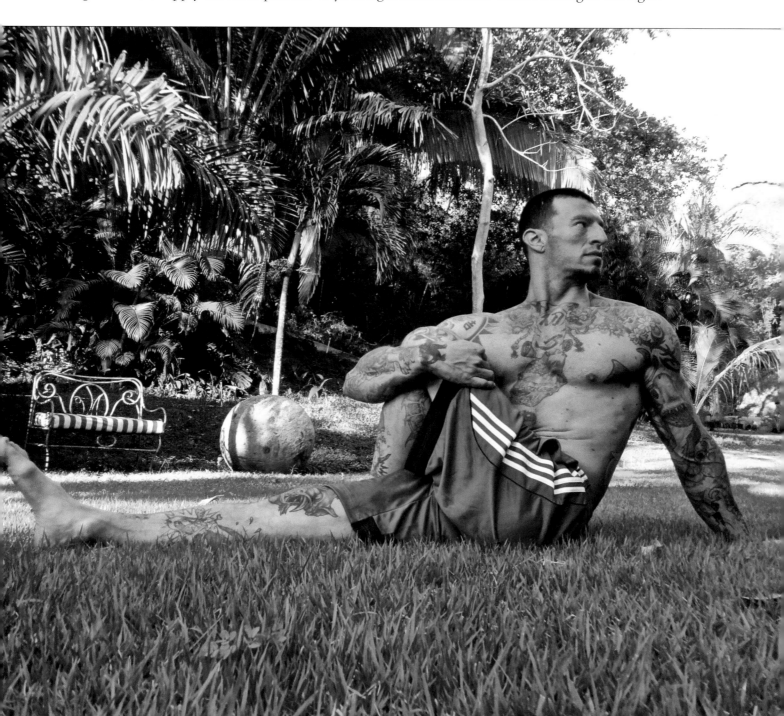

HIP FLEXORS STRETCH

The hip flexors are not the abs. However many people find it difficult to separate them during exercise. This is not an issue exclusive to beginners either; I've known many fit individuals who have trained for years who find it challenging to work their "lower" abs without excessive dependence on the hip flexors.

It makes sense; it's virtually impossible to separate them 100%. For these reasons, I feel it's important to include this stretch.

Start out at the bottom of a split-squat position with both knees bent to about 90 degrees. Your left leg should be in front of you with the foot flat on the floor. Your right knee should be beneath your hip, touching the ground as well. Now lean forward, keeping your torso up, bending the hip flexor and allowing your right knee to get farther behind you as you stretch. Hold for several breaths. Repeat on the other side.

Trainer Talk: For optimum stability, make sure to keep the glutes engaged. This will help you stretch the flexors, not just tilt the pelvis. Some find it more comfortable to keep a mat under their knee.

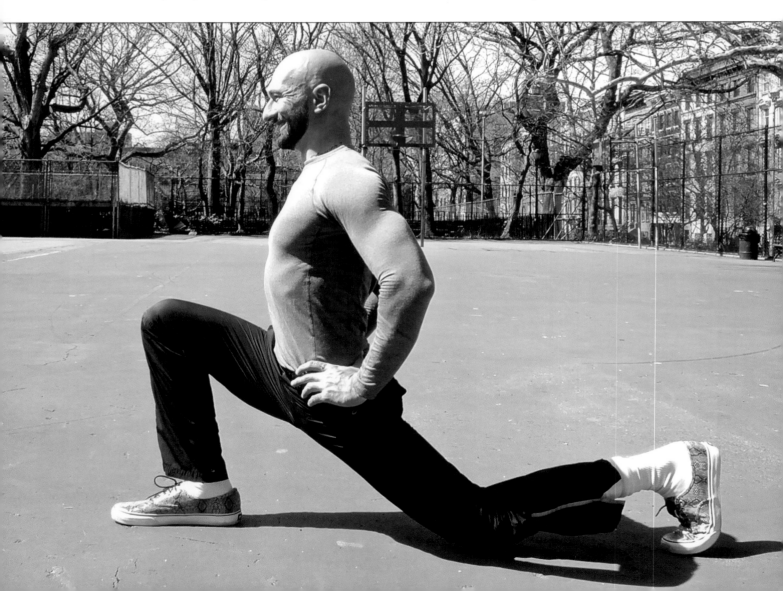

DEEP DOWN SQUAT

This is not technically an abs stretch, but it is one of my favorite stretches for overall mobility, health and wellness. The Deep Down Squat is exactly what it sounds like, however it is not done for reps; we just want to stay low and open up.

Begin with a standard bodyweight squat. When you get to the bottom, relax and "sit into it". Let your weight shift from your heels to your toes and side-to-side. Beginners may have a hard time keeping their heels down. After several breaths, your hips should begin to open and you should be able to get in a deeper squat. Improving range of motion could take twenty minutes, twenty weeks, or twenty months depending on circumstances. It's a process. Don't rush.

Though this stretch may feel unusual at first if you're new to stretching, it will ultimately be very relaxing in time. One can potentially stay in this position for hours on end.

Trainer Talk: The Deep Down Squat can be done every day, many times a day, for life. It may eventually become a comfortable resting pose.

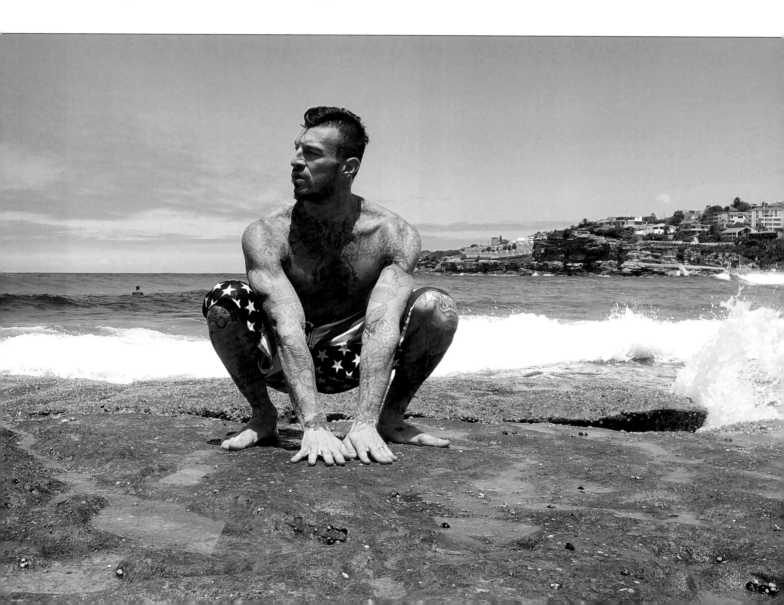

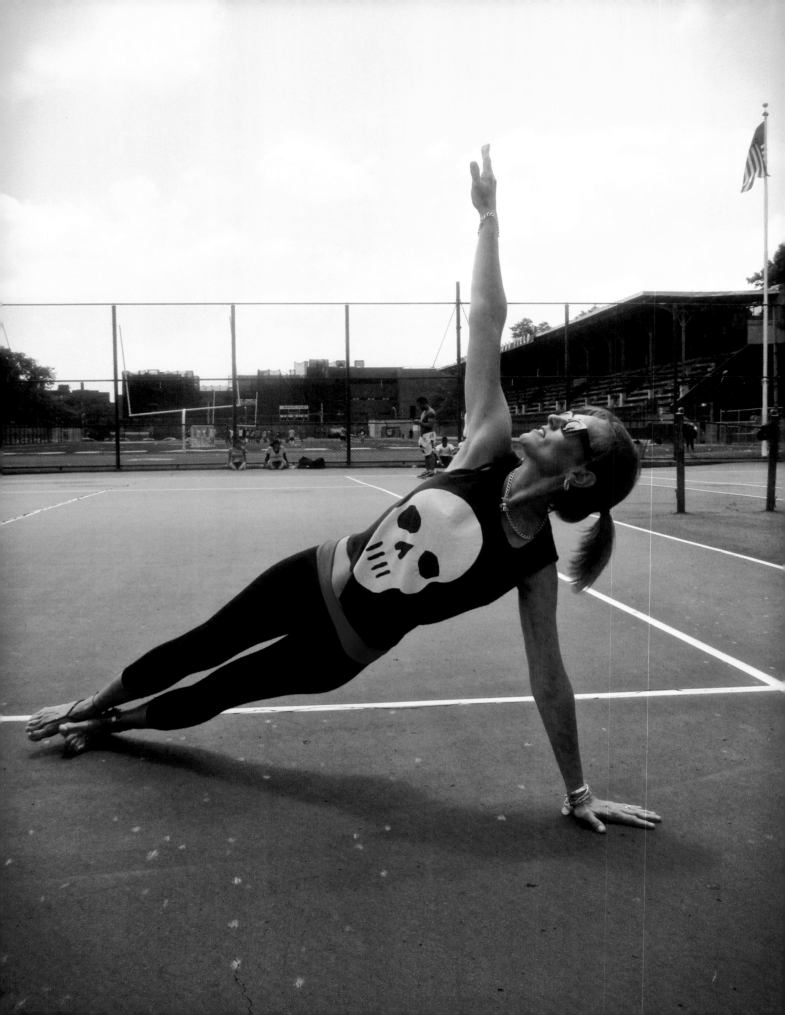

WORKOUTS

Fellow Brooklynite Mike Tyson famously remarked, "Everyone has a plan 'til they get punched in the face." Though it's good to have a layout, we must allow ourselves to adjust for what is actually happening in the moment.

It goes without saying that any abs-specific workout is meant to supplement, not replace, a full body strength training program. Don't just train your abs; you must squat, push and pull. I cannot be clearer than that. Yes, we will zone in on the abs in this chapter but full body training is a pre-requisite in this book.

When designing an abs program, be appropriate. Hit all areas. This is why the 80's fad of hundreds of crunches failed; it doesn't target the entire abdomen, just a small part of it again and again and again.

I encourage you work on your favorite exercises, but make sure to keep your program well rounded. When your body gets used to doing the same things repeatedly, it will get very good at those exercises, which will become less challenging, diminishing in effectiveness over time. It's important to mix it up in order to avoid physical and mental plateaus. Shock your system.

Here are some sample workouts, meant only to serve as guidelines. All of them can be done 3-5 times per week. Pay attention to intensity and body awareness. Be mindful of every rep. (Refer back to Chapter 12 Fundamentals Of Abdominal Strength Training for more on this subject.)

Take from these workouts what you wish. Train hard and have fun. Let's get Diamond-Cut!

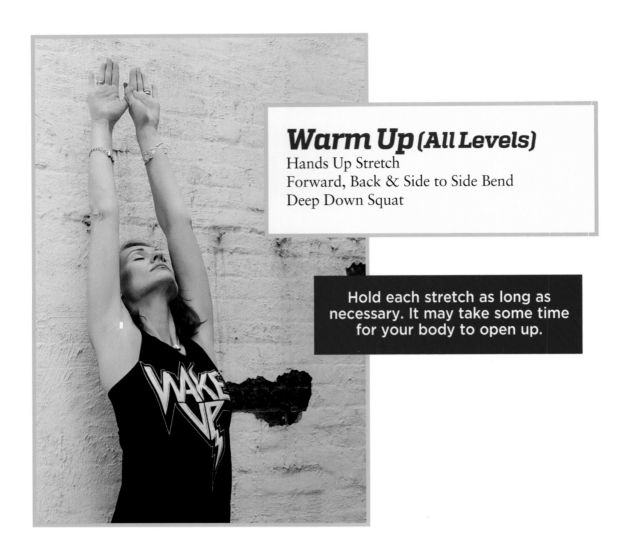

Warm Up (All Levels)
Hands Up Stretch
Forward, Back & Side to Side Bend
Deep Down Squat

Hold each stretch as long as necessary. It may take some time for your body to open up.

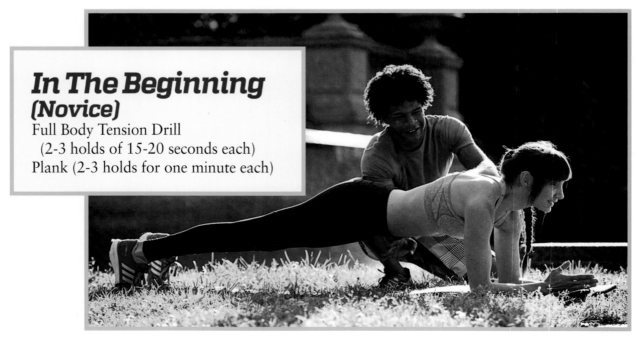

In The Beginning (Novice)
Full Body Tension Drill
 (2-3 holds of 15-20 seconds each)
Plank (2-3 holds for one minute each)

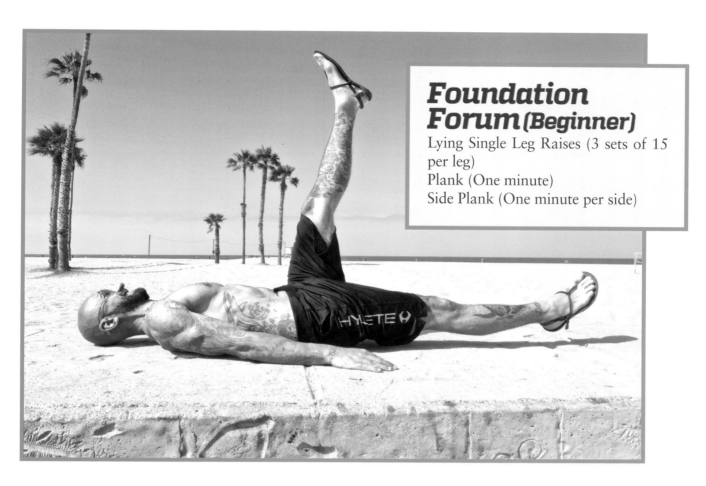

Foundation Forum (Beginner)

Lying Single Leg Raises (3 sets of 15 per leg)
Plank (One minute)
Side Plank (One minute per side)

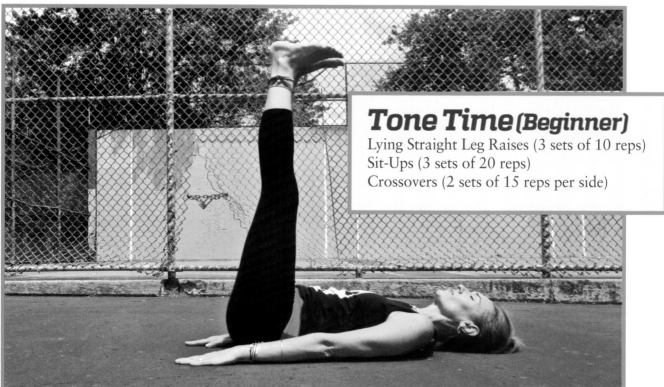

Tone Time (Beginner)

Lying Straight Leg Raises (3 sets of 10 reps)
Sit-Ups (3 sets of 20 reps)
Crossovers (2 sets of 15 reps per side)

Carve The Six (Intermediate)

Straight Arm/Straight Leg Crossovers (3 sets of 15 reps per side)
Grounded Wipers (3 sets of 20 reps)
Hanging Bicycles (30-60 seconds slow and controlled)

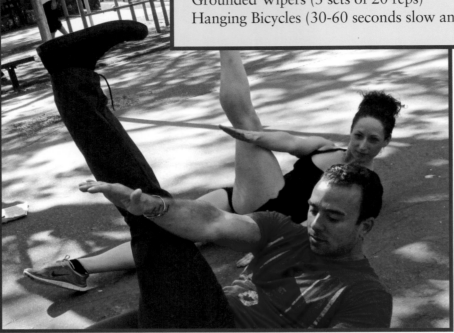

Burnout
(Intermediate)

N-Sit Until Failure
Hanging Knee Raises
  w/ a Twist (3 sets of 20 reps)
Jackknives (2 sets of 20 reps)
Plank Until Failure

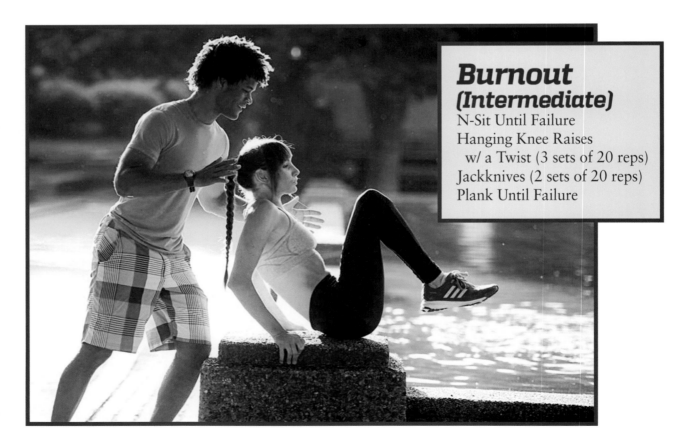

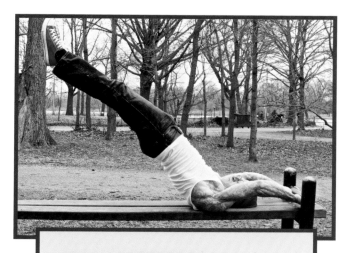

Shredding Season (Advanced)

L-Sit (One minute)
Washing Machines (3 sets of 20 reps)
Ab Wheel (4 sets of 5 reps)
Dragon Flag (2-3 sets of 5 reps)

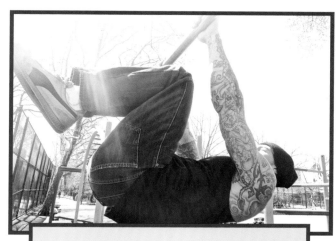

Abs Almighty (Advanced)

Hanging Leg Raises--Shins To Bar
  (3 sets of 15 reps)
Circles (3 sets of 20 reps)
Tuck Front Lever (30 second hold)
One Arm Flex Hang
  (20 second hold each side)

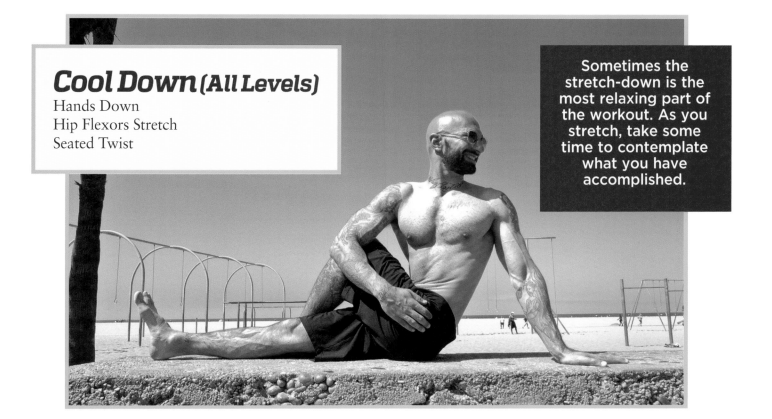

Cool Down (All Levels)

Hands Down
Hip Flexors Stretch
Seated Twist

Sometimes the stretch-down is the most relaxing part of the workout. As you stretch, take some time to contemplate what you have accomplished.

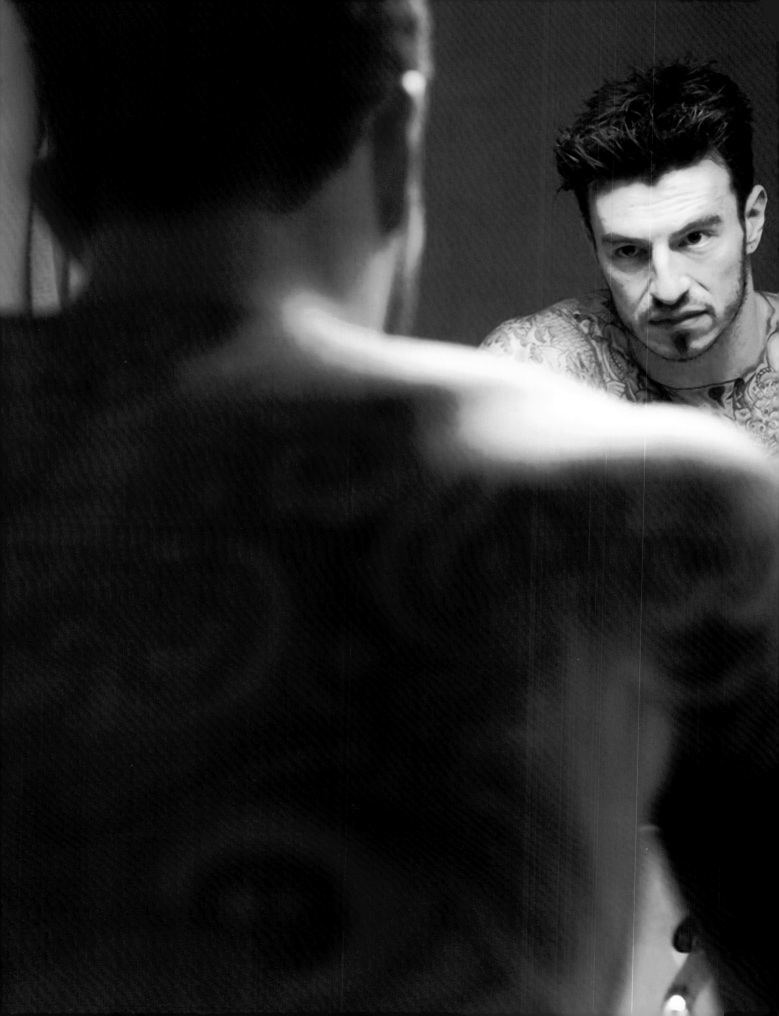

PART V

ABS & LIFESTYLE

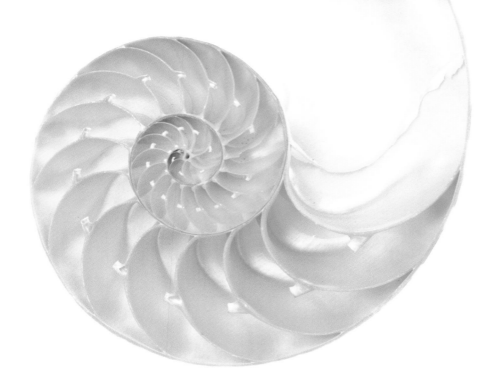

"The only way we can grow and get on in this world is to accept the fact we're not perfect and live accordingly."
–Ray Bradbury, from The Illustrated Man

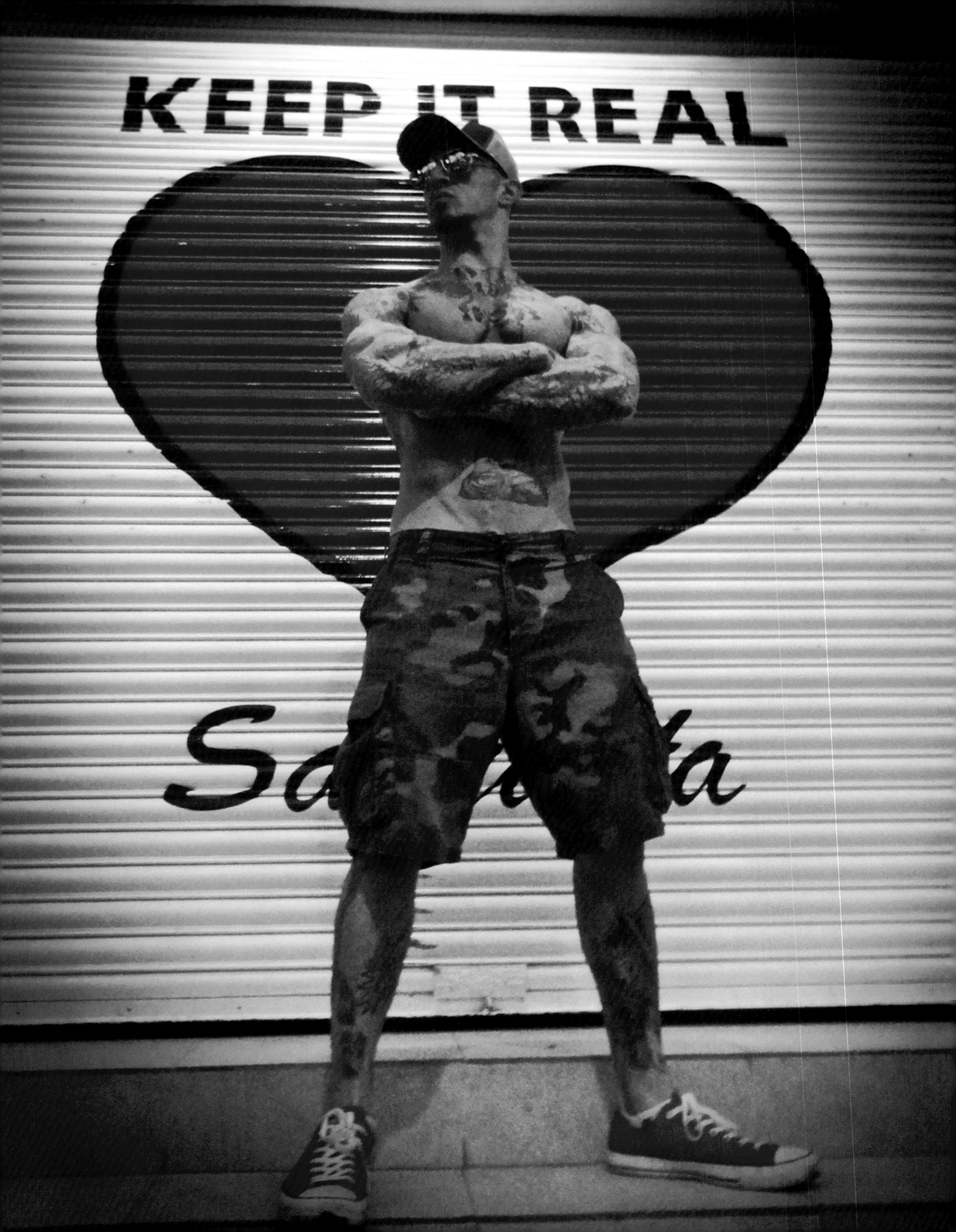
KEEP IT REAL

VIVA LA VIDA

Working hard is useless without enjoying your world, so eat the food, see the sights, love your lover, live the life. I am all about discipline, but let's keep everything in perspective.

Owning a rock-hard set of Diamond-Cut Abs is nice, but it will never be as important as family, experience, friendship or imagination. The pursuit of abs should improve your quality of life not take away from it.

Fitness in general should be enjoyed. Incorporating a workout program into your lifestyle should make you feel good not stressed out or deprived. Although we speak often of effort and accountability, it should never be at the expense of pleasure and fulfillment. There is room for both. You must find the balance.

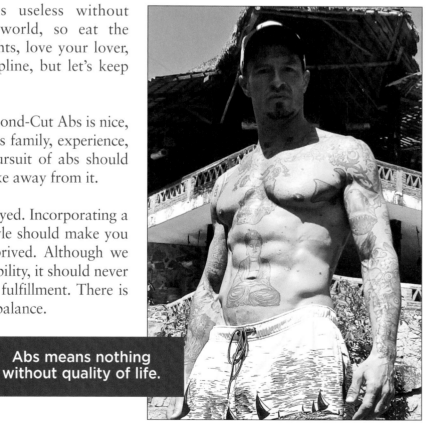

Abs means nothing without quality of life.

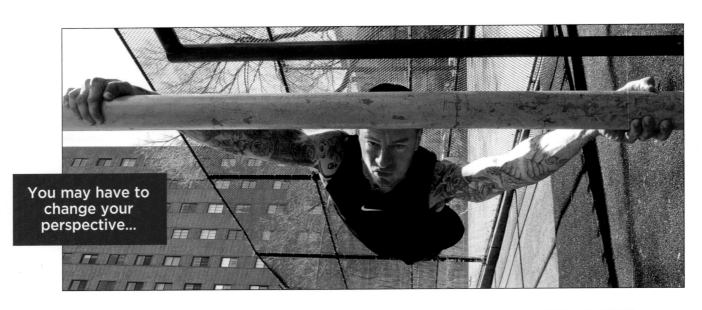

You may have to change your perspective...

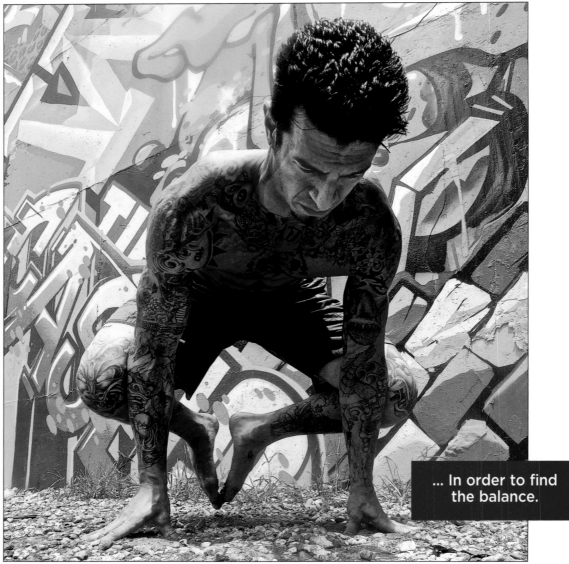

... In order to find the balance.

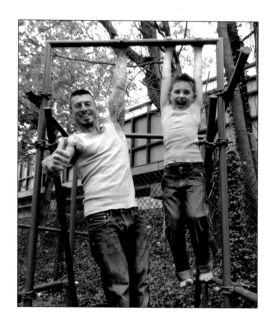

We can all stand to incorporate more movement into our lives. Get out of your car. Go for a jog. Take the stairs. We were built to move. Exercise isn't just healthy… it's a biological necessity! The human body is by far the most advanced, best designed and most mechanically sound workout gear there is—as the saying goes, use it or lose it!

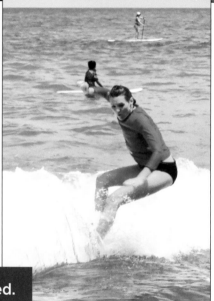

Yes, being goal-oriented has its merit, but I encourage a life-oriented approach to training. While it's true that any healthy individual can achieve the ripped six-pack of their dreams, we must focus on the process, not just the outcome. It's one step at a time and one rep at a time. Each day is its own and it's important to live in the present whether you're planting tomatoes or doing Jackknives. Each contributes to the end result but demands individual attention, for which you are greatly rewarded. Go with the flow and give each moment of your journey the respect it deserves.

We keep it life-oriented.

The Early Bird

We often focus on diet and exercise, while neglecting the importance of a good night's rest. You need sleep so your body can grow, repair, and get strong. The amount required is different for everybody. It can even change within the same individual depending on time of year, present lifestyle, energy expenditure and many other factors.

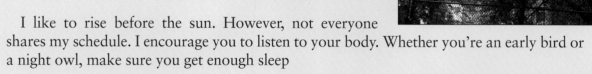

I like to rise before the sun. However, not everyone shares my schedule. I encourage you to listen to your body. Whether you're an early bird or a night owl, make sure you get enough sleep

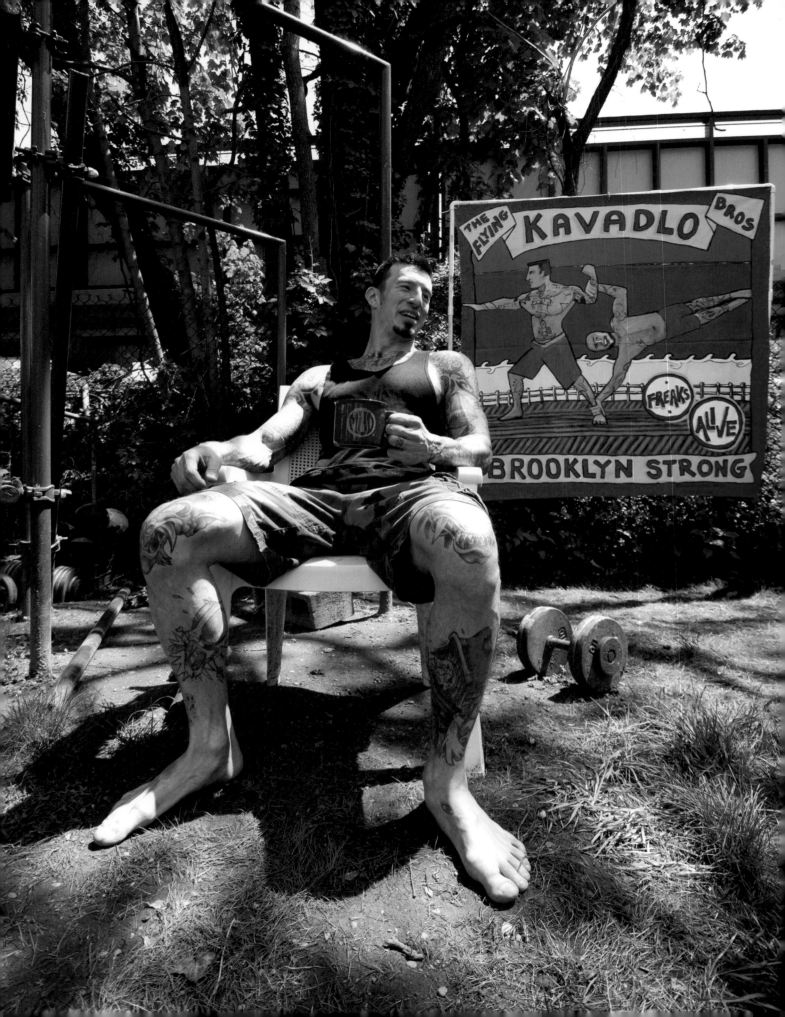

CHAPTER 22

THE MUD AND THE BLOOD AND THE BEER

It is possible to enjoy coffee, wine and beer and still maintain Diamond-Cut Abs. Not all potent potables are created equally.

I drink one cup of coffee with whole milk every morning. Like grains, animal products and fruit, there is a lot of conflicting "expert" opinion about coffee. Some say it has numerous health benefits, like improved athletic performance and increased fat loss; detractors speak of toxins and dehydration. Here's what we do know: Mankind has been enjoying coffee and tea for a long time, spanning cultures, continents and millennia. It's from the earth. I do not recommend adding any type of sugar (even honey, nectar or "raw" sugar) if you want abs, though. Many of the espresso inspired beverages sold at coffee chain restaurants tend to resemble desserts more than coffee, and should be treated as such. Always be aware of what you're putting in your body. Additionally, too much of almost anything is possible, even caffeine.

Alcohol is more controversial than coffee, and rightly so. I am generally fond of wine, but like ice cream (which I'm also fond of), I don't consume it every day. Whether you're drinking water or whiskey, like all foods, the quality of your beverage matters. I never understood how anyone could think that all wine is inherently bad. Very few foods are ever tended to with the amount of care as good wine. So much attention is paid to the grapes, the soil, even the rainfall. I wish everything I consumed was raised with the same attention to detail!

Like coffee consumption, wine intake has its friends and enemies. For everyone who says that the antioxidants in red wine are heart-healthy and help protect your blood vessels, others will accurately point out that too much alcohol of any kind can be harmful to your body.

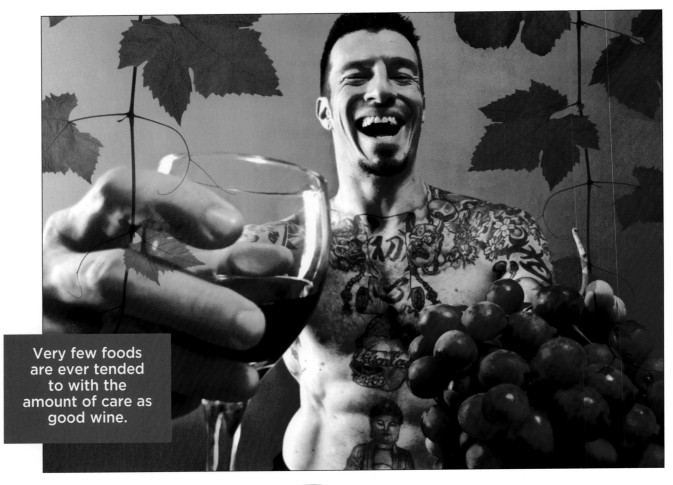

Very few foods are ever tended to with the amount of care as good wine.

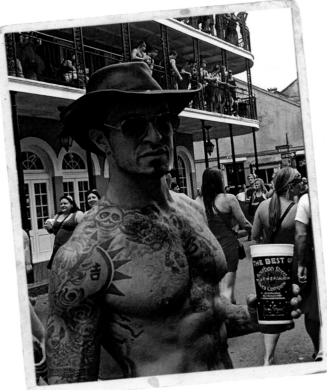

Liquor is harder to justify than wine. It is nutritionally barren and calorically dense. But the truth is, enjoying it sporadically will not necessarily destroy all the hard work you've done sculpting your abs. Other fitness professionals may take exception to my comparatively liberal views, but I stand by them. Obviously, too much alcohol is toxic and can ruin your life, but there is no reason a grown-up can't enjoy an occasional drink or two and still rock a ripped set of Diamond-Cut Abs. I do. If you are eating right 90% of the time and training hard, you've earned it, bub!

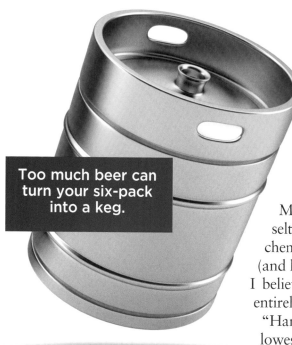

Too much beer can turn your six-pack into a keg.

Beer: It's packed with calories and will therefore pack on the pounds. Like eating too many chocolate kisses, onion bagels, or Boston cream pies, anything not metabolized can and will be stored as fat. Too much beer will turn your six-pack into a keg.

To me, mixed drinks are an even harder sell than beer. Most mixers like Margarita mix, cola and tonic (NOT seltzer or soda water) are loaded with sugar, sweeteners and chemicals. They are probably more detrimental to your abs (and health) than the booze itself. If you want washboard abs, I believe it's probably best to eliminate sugary mixed drinks entirely, or at the very least, to have extremely sparingly. "Hard" lemonades and ciders are the worst—they are the lowest quality alcohol combined with the lowest quality sugar. Stay away.

It's important to drink water consistently when enjoying any of the afore-mentioned beverages. While some of us are more impervi-ous to hangovers or coffee headaches than others, I rec-ommend that everybody have one glass of water for *every* beer, wine or spirit they consume, in addition to sev-eral glasses a day for general hydration purposes.

Adults make their own decisions. I am not here to tell you what to do or not to do. I simply want to promote

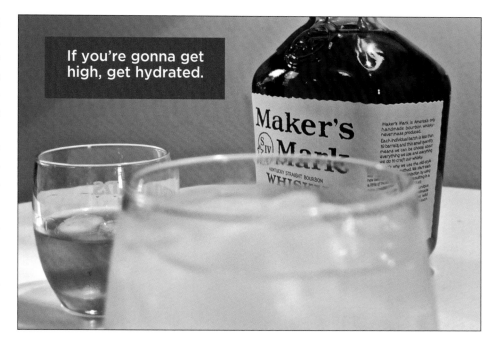

If you're gonna get high, get hydrated.

what I've viewed to be true regarding abs and health as objectively as possible. Often in the world of wellness, fear mongering tactics and absolutism trump life experience and common sense. Make up your own mind. As the saying goes: "All things in moderation... even moderation."

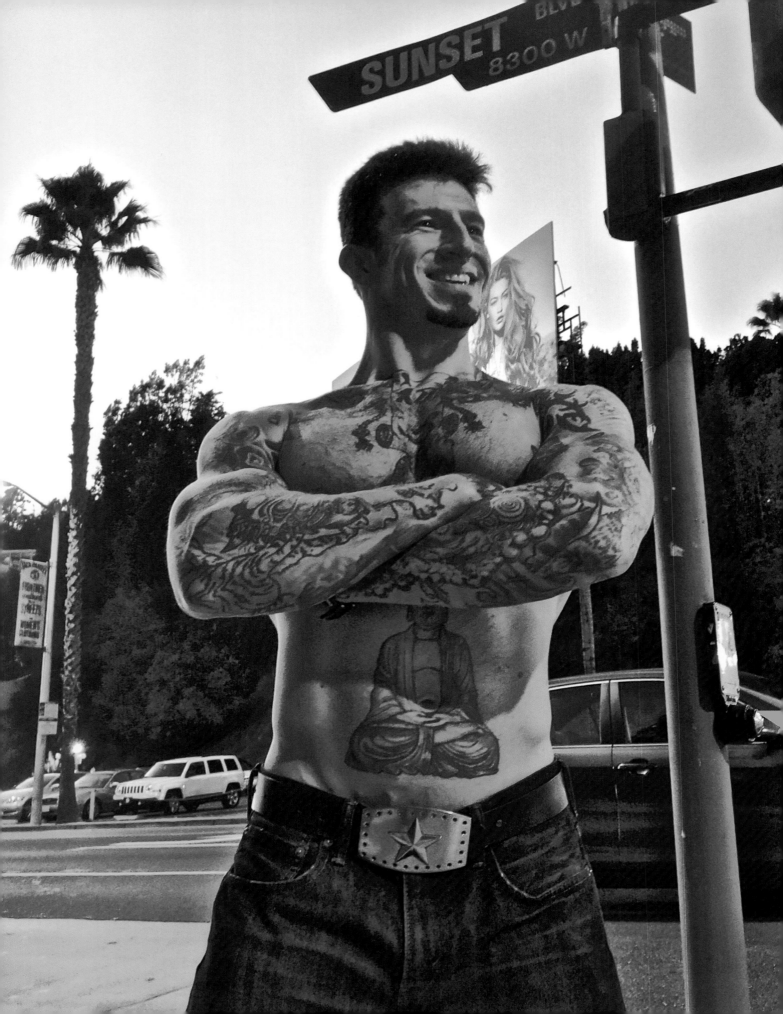

CHAPTER 23

SEASONS

On their 1968 album *Odyssey and Oracle*, the Zombies had their biggest hit ever with "Time Of The Season". Although they were singing about love, the phrase can easily be applied to our bodies in terms of the seasons' effects on our mood, metabolism, energy levels and even diet.

Consider this: if the Earth's rotation and revolution can move mountains over the centuries, then imagine what it can do to little ol' us. Ice caps melt. Tidal waves crash. Continents divide. We tiny mortals don't stand a chance.

Our physicality and emotions are dictated at least in part by the seasons. Our abs are no exception. In fact, nobody trains, eats or looks exactly the same in the summer as they do in the winter. Most of the photographs in this book were taken over the course of an entire year. The season's the reason! I wanted to show that the body changes throughout the year… just like everything else on the planet. I could have easily included only photos from the summer, or after fasting for a week, but that would not have been very honest. Think back to Chapter 1. My goal with this book is to tell the truth, even when it's not what most people want to hear.

In the dark, chilly days of winter, many of us get run down. With less daylight, we stay indoors and tend not to move around as much. We eat more and expend less energy. As mammals with the instinct to bulk up as temperatures drop, our biology tells us to gain weight just like a bear's tells it to hibernate. Even dear Mother Nature is an accomplice as heavier, starchier foods come into season. That's the way it goes. Showing restraint at the dinner table can be difficult this time of year. For some people, it even takes extra effort just to work out! But it's worth it. Don't miss out on training just because it's cold.

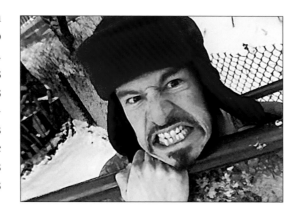

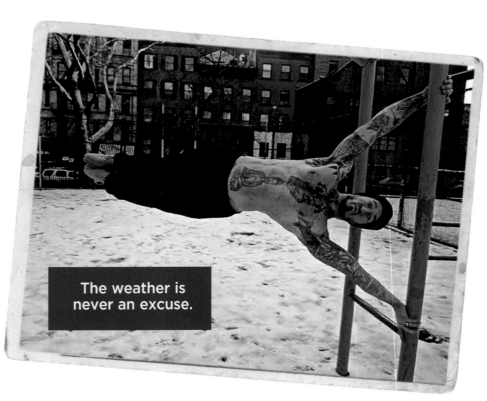

The weather is never an excuse.

We've grown soft as a species in general, enjoying things like sitting, driving and climate control a little too much. It's good to experience the elements. I learned to love winter once I embraced it.

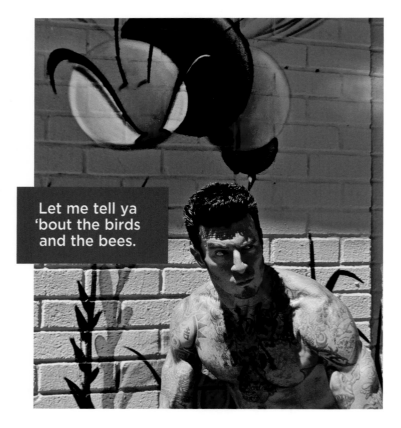

Let me tell ya 'bout the birds and the bees.

Unlike the winter months, just about everybody enjoys being outside in the springtime. Flowers blooming, bees buzzing, birds chirping. When spring fever is in the air, even the laziest tend to, at least temporarily, get up and move. Naturally, spring is the time of year when even people who were negligent about their training all winter, want to play catch-up by the summer. This is not usually realistic.

Who doesn't love springtime? Our moods improve in the sunshine. We feel warm and alive and everyone wants to take their clothes off. Spring is a great time to capitalize on these feelings. Train hard and have fun.

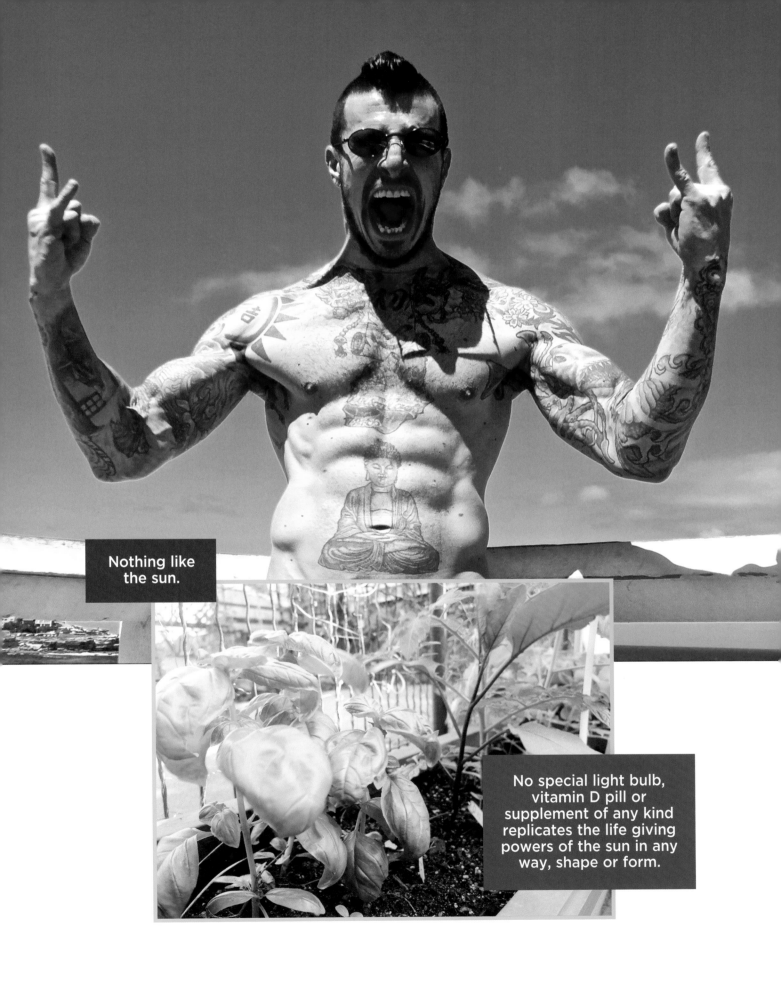

Nothing like the sun.

No special light bulb, vitamin D pill or supplement of any kind replicates the life giving powers of the sun in any way, shape or form.

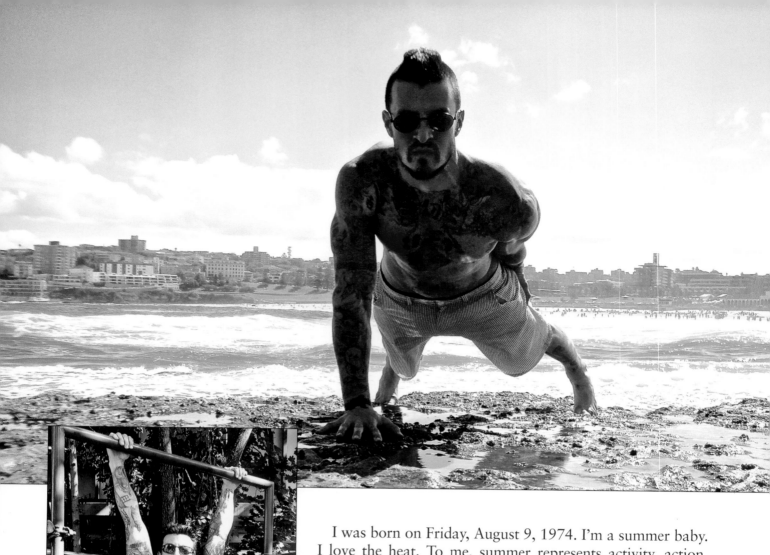

The Pumpkin Knee Raise is a fantastic autumn exercise.

I was born on Friday, August 9, 1974. I'm a summer baby. I love the heat. To me, summer represents activity, action, intensity and passion. I enjoy training in the summertime.

By now, we understand the role of energy expenditure and food intake in the path towards Diamond-Cut Abs. In those hot months, we tend to move around a lot more. Exercise feels natural as the body is already warmed up. Go forward with it.

Plus, fruits and vegetables are live, luscious and available! Berries, melons and greens are in season and we are biologically craving them. I practically live at the farmers market in the summertime. I grow my own herbs, tomatoes and peppers as heavy, greasy, starchy foods lose their appeal. Summer abs is natural.

Being from New York, I used to take autumn's elegant beauty for granted. As a kid, it just meant back-to-school. But when I got older and travelled the country, I began to appreciate what a truly wonderful season it is, especially after visiting

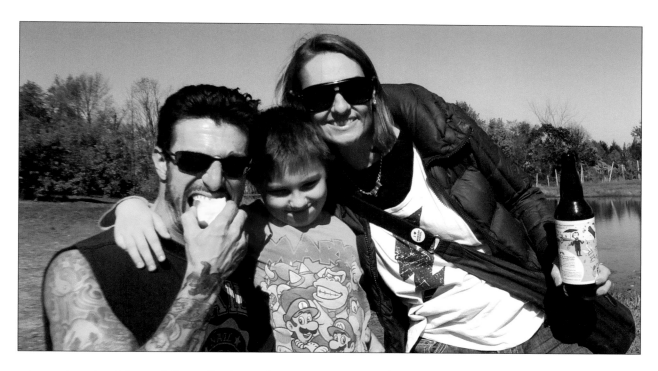

places that don't have fall at all. Now I love it. Autumn is the bridge from summer into winter. The leaves change colors and fall from the trees. We can play in the leaves. Blueberries give way to starchier produce, like squash and pumpkins. I love my summer berries, but as the saying goes, change is good. Autumn is change.

And ultimately, that's why you're holding this book: to change. Accept that for your abs to change, you must change yourself. I understand that we are often told the opposite. Just this morning, I viewed a clip of a reputable TV doctor explaining how a "natural" pill will burn fat with "No exercise, No diet, No effort". That's literally what the clip said. It makes me sad when such foolishness is perpetuated as fact. Like the TV doctor, I believe that, yes, we can all burn fat and have a set of indestructable abdominals, but unlike the pitchman, I make no secret that *it will take effort and effort takes time.*

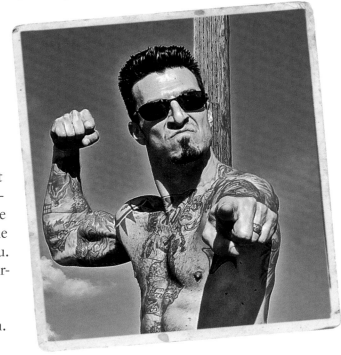

I consider the practice of owning Diamond-Cut Abs to be a journey. And like any practice or discipline, your involvement will change throughout the seasons of your life. It truly is an odyssey. Go with the flow. Life and fitness should be enjoyed; it's up to you. Accept change, but never be afraid to create it yourself.

Nothing changes but the changes. Make it happen.

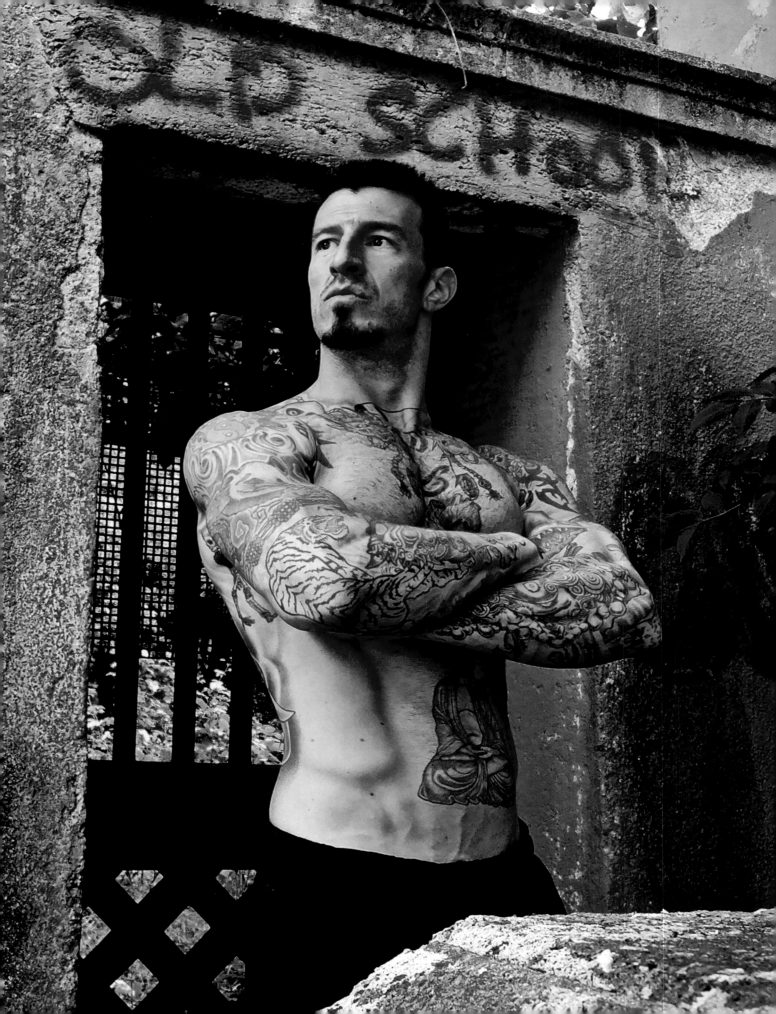

ABOUT THE AUTHOR

Danny Kavadlo is one of the world's foremost authorities on calisthenics, nutrition and personal training. He is known for his minimalist philosophy, simple approach and motivational talents.

Mr. Kavadlo is the author of *Everybody Needs Training: Proven Success Secrets For The Professional Fitness Trainer* and is a Lead Instructor for *Dragon Door's Progressive Calisthenics Certification*. He has been featured in the *NY Times, Men's Fitness* and is a regular contributor to *Bodybuilding.com*.

Danny's been practicing strength training and calisthenics for almost thirty years and has been obsessed with abs for most of that time. He lives in Brooklyn, NY with his wife Jennifer and son Wilson. They enjoy food, traveling and the being in the sun.

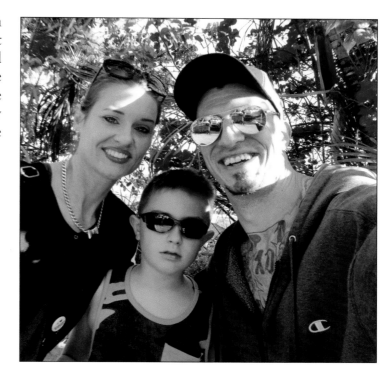

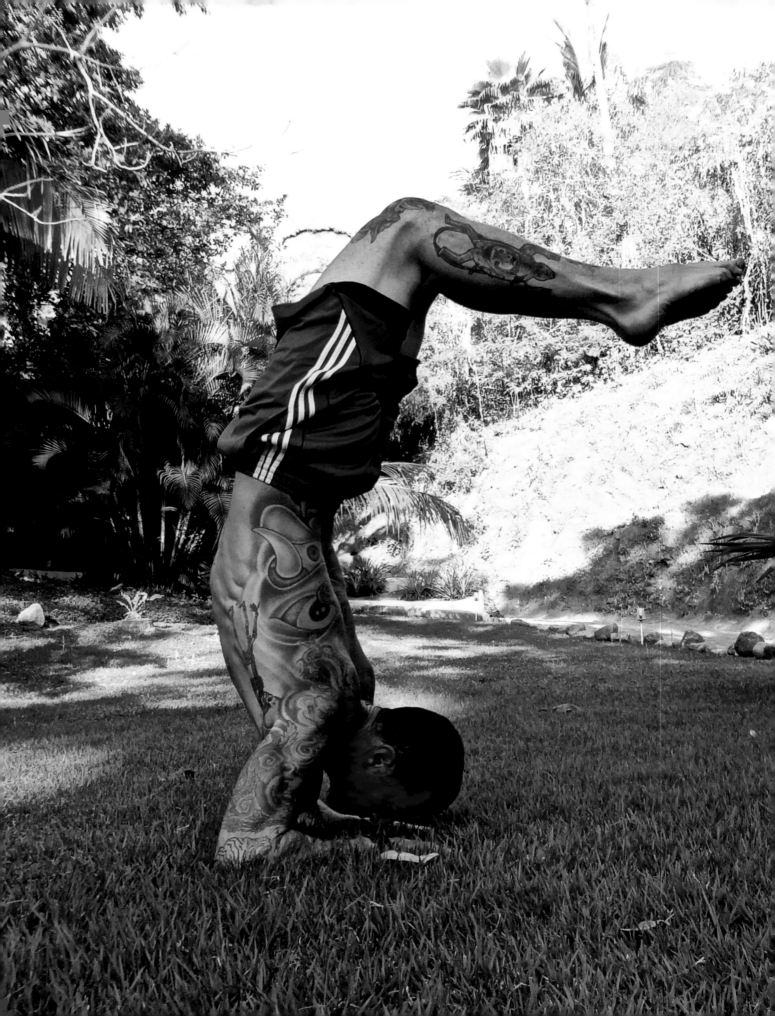

GRATITUDE

To my wife Jennifer, you've held my hand and walked side-by-side through the fire with me for almost ten years. No one has ever made me feel alive like you do. Baby, what can I say? You are the one. I fucking love you to death.

Wilson it was you who told me to write a book that had exercises in it. Thanks for the advice. You are my biggest inspiration and my greatest sense of joy. Of all the things I've ever accomplished, I'm most proud of you.

To my parents, Rosalie and Carl, thank you for standing by me through the best and worst decisions of my life without judgment. You guys have shown me nothing but love and support. I just hope I show it back.

My brother Al: You are my trainer, editor, photographer, model, motivator and over-all partner in crime. But above all you are my best friend. The words "thank you" do not come close.

My brother Jesse: I could not be the man I am today without having had you in my life. Thank you for giving me someone to look up to as a kid.

Thanks to my dear friends Mike Anderson and Matthew Mangiaracina. It brings me great joy to still have you guys in my life. Nuthin' but love, brothers.

Tremendous thanks to John Du Cane, Dennis Armstrong, Rose Widell, Tammy Drury, Allison Olson, Mumtaz Walli-Ware and the entire crew at Dragon Door. It is a privilege to be associated with the best of the best. Here's to our continued success together!

Gigantic gratitude to Paul "Coach" Wade for bringing the old school calisthenic methods to the forefront, while revolutionizing the industry at the same time. But on a personal level, I'd like to thank the Coach for his support and belief in me. Coach Wade, I hope to thank you in person one day.

It's an honor to have Derek Brigham from dbrigham.com design this work. The man is a visual genius. Thanks for making my words look amazing, Big D!

Mad love and thanks to my entire Progressive Calisthenics family including: Adrienne Harvey, Fredrik Hogstrom, Chunhua Yang, Robert Rimoczi, Moritz Rammensee, Steven Graves, Adam Von Rothfelder, Jack Arnow, Adrian Harrington, Lyall Rowan, Angelo Gala, Beth Andrews, Steven Low, Anders Randlin, Benji Williford, Nick Kenon, Tanner Hubscher, Chris Garay, Laura Robertson, Andrew Read, Shannon Scullin, Matt Beecroft, James McConnell, Alby Owens, Martjin Bos, Logan Christopher and every PCC all over the world who ever stood tall and took on The Century! Thanks to all of you—the posse's gettin' bigger!

Thanks the following for coming through last minute for me with some world-class photos: My good friend and the Metro/DC area's #1 trainer Errick McAdams (www.empt.us), group fitness guru Slywia Wiesenberg (www.ToniqueFitness.com), the dynamic duo of Angelo Grinceri & Rosalia Chann (www.CouplesCalisthenics.com), my man Kevin Richardson (www.NaturallyIntense.net), the amazing team of Rick Richards & Jasmine Brooks (www.FitBeyondLimitsPersonalTraining.com) & the West Coast's newest rising star of strength and mobility Grace Menendez. Thank you for helping make this book look so damn good!

Special thanks to Jennie Willink, Liz Gilbert, Rosally Sapla, Josh Murphy, Mike Gibson, Jeff Bodnar, Phil LeDesma, Ronnie Love, Tony Ebanks, Eric Berggmann, Eric Reyelt, Rob Severiano, Trainer Steve, Peter Ngo, Nader Freij, Tom Legath, Mike Spiegel, Tony Hamoui, Raul Robinson, Jose Perez, Cisco Alfonseca, Terence Gore, Kalvin Dukes, Jose Mota, Kelly Jo Johnson, Maria Simone, Alfred DiGrazia, Jason Quick, Steven Ram, Mike Fitch, Mike Wilson, Dana James, Emma Goldsmith, John Gaczewski, Arlene Patruno, Randy Humola, Edward Anthony, James Young, Daniel Lucas, Antonio Sini, Keith Payne, Andrew Speer, Albert Matheny, Ryan Hopkins & Eric Planas. You guys have helped me more than you know and I am grateful.

I am eternally thankful to all my friends, fans and followers from all over the world. Thank you to everyone who's read one word I've written, looked at any of my photos or commented, positive or negative, on anything I've ever done. Keep on spreading the word!

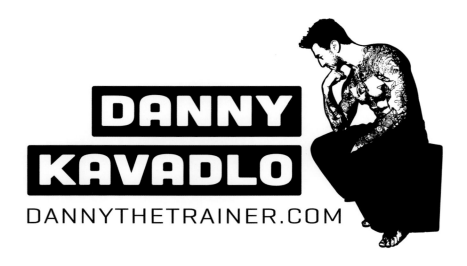

DANNY KAVADLO
DANNYTHETRAINER.COM

To my brothers and sisters in the calisthenics community and every single hard working trainer out there: Thank you for being down with the cause and promoting the medicine of movement! HELLYEAH!

When all is said and done, I believe I owe thanks to everyone I ever met in my life, as they all contributed to exactly what you see today. I wouldn't change a thing.

Keep the dream alive my friends,

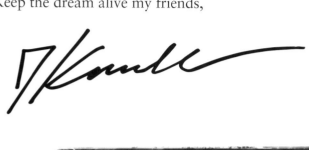

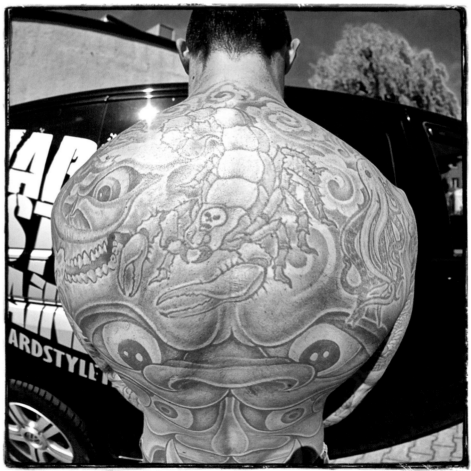

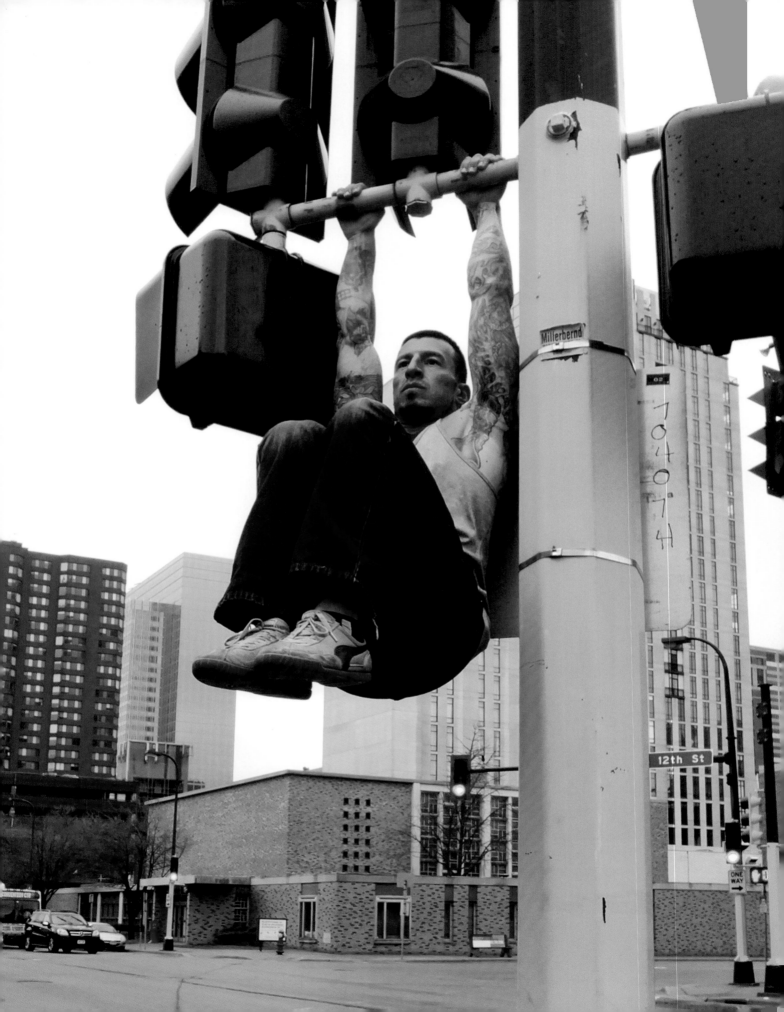

INDEX OF EXERCISES

— Exercise Your Demons —

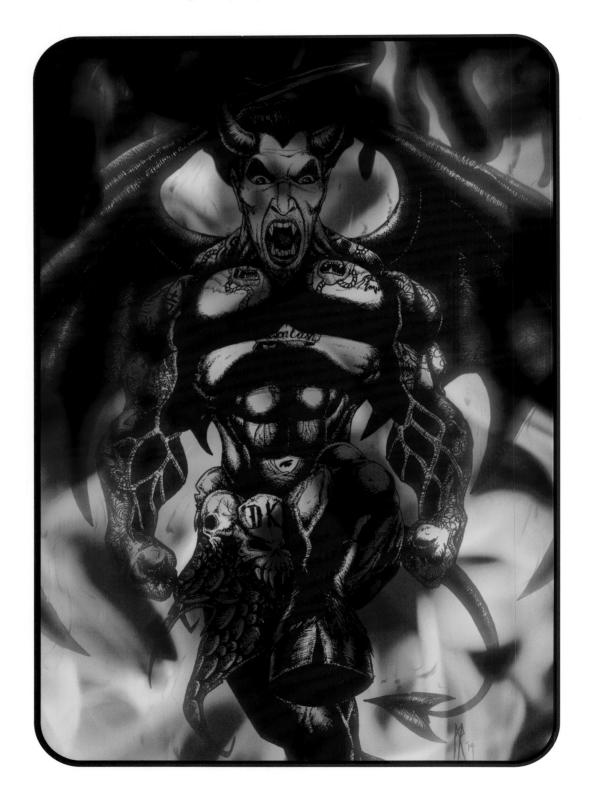

Most folk who embark on a career as a trainer, do so initially out of a personal passion for fitness and a strong desire to help other achieve results. Be it weight loss, conditioning, strength gains, flexibility or enhanced performance.

But a passion for working out and an earnest desire to help others—alone—does not a successful personal trainer make. The sad fact is that the turn over rate for personal trainers after one year is over 80%. Why? It's almost always because the trainer didn't have a proper understanding of the BUSINESS of being a fitness professional.

The bottom line is that without the appropriate success blueprint, the most skilled and knowledgeable personal trainer is usually doomed to failure. Unfortunately, until now, there has been no such battle-tested blueprint available either to the novice trainer or the professional struggling to stay alive. Now, however that's all changed, thanks to Danny Kavadlo's Everybody Needs Training. Follow the hard-earned wisdom within these pages and failure will no longer be an option.

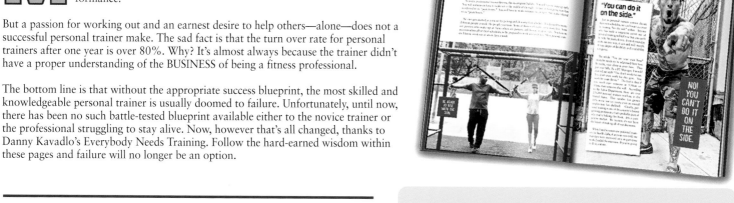

"*Everybody Needs Training* is quite 'something.' I don't think I have ever seen this kind of depth in the field. It's both obvious and 'wow' as you read it. Amazing stuff. It fills a gap in the community that, frankly, surprises me no one has really filled."—DAN JOHN, author, *Never Let Go*

"Danny Kavadlo has personally helped me become a more successful trainer and coach. I cannot recommend Everybody Needs Training enough. It's the best book I've ever seen on the subject of being a professional trainer."
—ADEL GABER, World Class Trainer & 3-Time Olympic Wrestling Coach

"*Everybody Needs Training* is a solid collection of tried-and-true best practices that can help personal trainers on any level reach their full potential in their chosen field."—ROLANDO GARCIA, RKC II, CK-FMS

"*Everybody Needs Training* is a must-read for every personal trainer wanting to take it to the next level, and everyone who has ever dreamed of becoming a personal trainer. This book allows you to get inside the genius PT mind of Danny Kavadlo, a master of his craft, speaking off the cuff to you about training—priceless!"—ERRICK MCADAMS, Personal Trainer, Model, Fitness Personality

Good for any profession or business

"I'm not a trainer, but took Danny and Al's PCC Class. This is a great book for anyone going into business as either an employee or owner, whether a fitness trainer or any other kind of business. I'm a lawyer, and I'm thinking about making it required reading for my newly hired lawyers. Good practical advice, with the focus on the customer, which is a focus that seems to be lost these days. Easy reading, but pithy, with lots of great tips and ideas, with an excellent overriding theme. Oh yea -- well written too!"— Mark Walker, McAllen, Texas

"Christmas wishes DO come true....Danny Kavadlo has written a training book! Imagine if you could squeeze all the hard-earned wisdom, secrets and tactics of one of the world's hottest personal trainers between the covers of a beautifully illustrated tell-all manual, and you have imagined *Everybody Needs Training*.

Like Danny himself, this groundbreaking book is incredibly smart, brutally honest, laugh-out-loud funny, and totally out of left field…if you train others (casually or professionally), want a career training others, or if you just love the now-famous "Kavadlo approach" to getting in shape, you owe it to yourself to grab a copy of this masterpiece. I cannot recommend it highly enough."
—PAUL WADE, author of *Convict Conditioning*

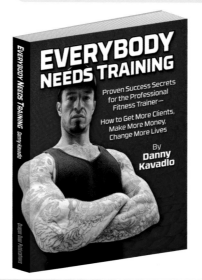

Everybody Needs Training
Proven Success Secrets for the Professional Fitness Trainer—How to Get More Clients, Make More Money, Change More Lives
By Danny Kavadlo
#B72 $34.95
eBook $19.95
Paperback 8.5 x 11   216 pages
253 photos

Beginner   Mid-Level   Advanced

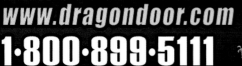

The Best Training Resolution You Can Make: Log Yourself—All Year Long!

The Fastest Way to Make Physical Progress a Guarantee—Besides Dedicated, Skillful Practice—Is to Keep a Training Log

We've all heard the phrase 'the spirit is willing but the flesh is weak'. And never was this more true than in the quest for strength!

So, what are the two golden keys, or secrets to bending the flesh to the spirit's desire?

The first secret is the system—and the system is dedicated, organized application over time. And in the hard world of strength that means keeping track of your goals and measuring your progress. When it comes to serious training, you keep a log or you fail. The sins of sloppiness, haphazardness, laziness and disorganization lay waste to our dreams of physical achievement—and sabotage the best intentions to beat our flesh into righteous steel. We invite you to exorcize the demons of weakness from your flesh—with a "religious" dedication to tracking and measuring—*Convict Conditioning* style.

The second secret for strength success is inspiration. In this stunning companion to his bestselling bodyweight exercise masterpieces, Convict Conditioning author Paul Wade, goes far, far beyond the traditional log book—by delivering a bucket-load of inspiring stories and jewel-like training tips to push you forward in your quest for ever-greater strength.

This book is the first-ever training log designed specifically for bodyweight athletes. Other logs are structured to contain sections where you detail the amount of weight you used, the type of equipment or machine you worked out on, even what your heart-rate was and what vitamins you took today. You won't find any of this distracting information in this log. It's a log for pure, unadulterated, hardcore bodyweight training. We provide the inspiration and the structure—you provide the perspiration and bloody-mindedness to seize the plan and make it happen.

There is a window of opportunity awaiting you. The strength gains that have continued to elude you can finally be yours. That window of opportunity lies within these pages and within your heart. Bring it!

By far the best log book we have seen, frankly, is **Paul Wade's *Convict Conditioning Ultimate Bodyweight Training Log***. But don't think that you have to use it just for your bodyweight work. It'll serve just as well to document your progress with kettlebells, martial arts or any other practice.

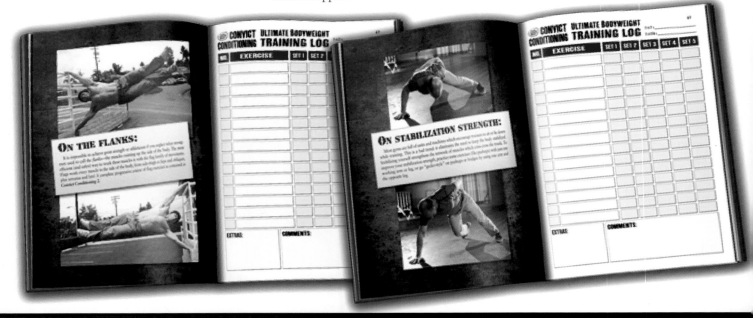

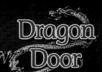

Reader Praise for Convict Conditioning Ultimate Bodyweight Training Log

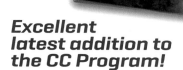

Above and Beyond!

"Not JUST a log book. TONS of great and actually useful info. I really like to over complicate programming and data entries at times. And honestly, All one has to do is fill in the blanks... Well that and DO THE WORK. Great product."
—Noel Price, Chicagoland, IL

A unique training log

"This log book is one of a kind in the world. It is the only published body weight exclusive training log I have personally seen. It is well structured and provides everything for a log book in a primarily body weight oriented routine. The book is best integrated with the other books in the convict conditioning series however has enough information to act as a stand alone unit. It is a must have for anyone who is a fan of the convict conditioning series or is entering into calisthenics." —Carter D., Cambridge, Canada

Excellent Companion to Convict Conditioning 1 & 2

"This is an amazing book! If you are a fan of Convict Conditioning (1 & 2) you need to get this training log. If you are preparing for the Progressive Calisthenics Certification then it's a must-have!!! The spiral bound format is a huge improvement over the regular binding and it makes it that much more functional for use in the gym. Great design, amazing pictures and additional content! Once again - Great job Dragon Door!"
—Michael Krivka, RKC Team Leader, Gaithersburg, MD

Excellent latest addition to the CC Program!

"A terrific book to keep you on track and beyond. Thank you again for this incredible series!"
—Joshua Hatcher, Holyoke, MA

Calling this a Log Book is Selling it Short

"I thought, what is the big deal about a logbook! Seriously mistaken. It is a work of art and with tips on each page that would be a great book all by itself. Get it. It goes way beyond a log book...the logging part of this book is just a bonus. You must have this!"—Jon Engum, Brainerd, MN

The Ultimate Bodyweight Conditioning

"I have started to incorporate bodyweight training into my strength building when I am not going to the gym. At the age of 68, after 30 years in the gym the 'Convict Conditioning Log' is going to be a welcome new training challenge."
—William Hayden, Winter Park, FL

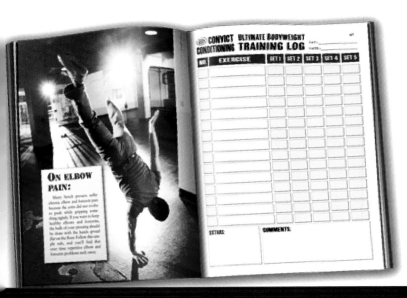

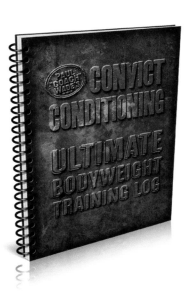

Convict Conditioning Ultimate Bodyweight Training Log

By Paul "Coach" Wade
#B67 $29.95
eBook $19.95

Paperback (spiral bound) 6 x 9
290 pages 175 photos

Beginner Mid-Level Advanced

How Do YOU Stack Up Against These 6 Signs of a TRUE Physical Specimen?

According to Paul Wade's *Convict Conditioning* you earn the right to call yourself a 'true physical specimen' if you can perform the following:

1. AT LEAST one set of 5 one-arm pushups each side—with the ELITE goal of 100 sets each side

2. AT LEAST one set of 5 one-leg squats each side—with the ELITE goal of 2 sets of 50 each side

3. AT LEAST a single one-arm pullup each side—with the ELITE goal of 2 sets of 6 each side

4. AT LEAST one set of 5 hanging straight leg raises—with the ELITE goal of 2 sets of 30

5. AT LEAST one stand-to-stand bridge—with the ELITE goal of 2 sets of 30

6. AT LEAST a single one-arm handstand pushup on each side— with the ELITE goal of 1 set of 5

Well, how DO you stack up?

Chances are that whatever athletic level you have achieved, there are some serious gaps in your OVERALL strength program. Gaps that stop you short of being able to claim status as a truly accomplished strength athlete.

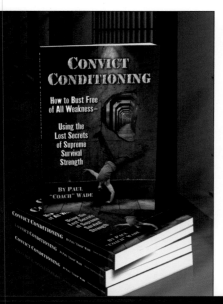

The good news is that—in *Convict Conditioning*—Paul Wade has laid out a brilliant 6-set system of 10 progressions which allows you to master these elite levels.

And you could be starting at almost any age and in almost in any condition...

Paul Wade has given you the keys—ALL the keys you'll ever need— that will open door, after door, after door for you in your quest for supreme physical excellence. Yes, it will be the hardest work you'll ever have to do. And yes, 97% of those who pick up *Convict Conditioning*, frankly, won't have the guts and the fortitude to make it. But if you make it even half-way through **Paul's Progressions**, you'll be stronger than almost anyone you encounter. Ever.

Here's just a small taste of what you'll get with *Convict Conditioning*:

Can you meet these 5 benchmarks of the *truly powerful*?... Page 1

The nature and the art of real strength... Page 2

Why mastery of *progressive calisthenics* is the ultimate secret for building maximum raw strength... Page 2

A dozen one-arm handstand pushups without support— anyone? Anyone?... Page 3

How to rank in a powerlifting championship—*without ever training with weights*... Page 4

Calisthenics as a hardcore strength training technology... Page 9

Spartan "300" calisthenics at the Battle of Thermopolylae... Page 10

How to cultivate the perfect body—the Greek and Roman way... Page 10

The difference between "old school" and "new school" calisthenics... Page 15

The role of prisons in preserving the older systems... Page 16

Strength training as a primary survival strategy... Page 16

The 6 basic benefits of bodyweight training... Pages 22—27

Why calisthenics are the *ultimate* in functional training... Page 23

The value of cultivating *self-movement*—rather than *object-movement*... Page 23

The *real* source of strength—it's not your *muscles*... Page 24

One crucial reason why a lot of convicts deliberately avoid weight-training... Page 24

How to progressively strengthen your joints over a lifetime—and even heal old joint injuries... Page 25

Why "authentic" exercises like pullups are so perfect for strength and power development... Page 25

Bodyweight training for quick physique perfection... Page 26

How to normalize and regulate your body fat levels—with bodyweight training only... Page 27

Why weight-training and the psychology of overeating go hand in hand... Page 27

The best approach for rapidly strengthening your whole body is this... Page 30

This is the most important and revolutionary feature of *Convict Conditioning*.... Page 33

A jealously-guarded system for going from puny to powerful— when your life may depend on the speed of your results... Page 33

The 6 "Ultimate" Master Steps—only a handful of athletes in the whole world can correctly perform them all. Can you?... Page 33

How to Forge Armor-Plated Pecs and Steel Triceps... Page 41

Why the pushup is the *ultimate* upper body exercise—and better than the bench press... Page 41

How to effectively bulletproof the vulnerable rotator cuff

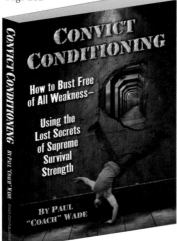

Beginner   Mid-Level   Advanced

Convict Conditioning

How to Bust Free of All Weakness—Using the Lost Secrets of Supreme Survival Strength

By Paul "Coach" Wade
#B41 $39.95
eBook $19.95

Paperback 8.5 x 11   320 pages
191 photos, charts and illustrations

Dragon Door Customer Acclaim for Paul Wade's *Convict Conditioning*

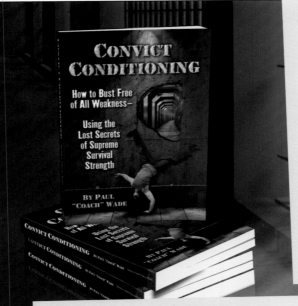

A Strength Training Guide That Will Never Be Duplicated!

"I knew within the first chapter of reading this book that I was in for something special and unique. The last time I felt this same feeling was when reading *Power to the People!* To me this is the Body Weight equivalent to Pavel's masterpiece.

Books like this can never be duplicated. Paul Wade went through a unique set of circumstances of doing time in prison with an 'old time' master of calisthenics. Paul took these lessons from this 70 year old strong man and mastered them over a period of 20 years while 'doing time'. He then taught these methods to countless prisoners and honed his teaching to perfection.

I believe that extreme circumstances like this are what it takes to create a true masterpiece. I know that 'masterpiece' is a strong word, but this is as close as it gets. No other body weight book I have read (and I have a huge fitness library)...comes close to this as far as gaining incredible strength from body weight exercise.

Just like Power to the People, I am sure I will read this over and over again...mastering the principles that Paul Wade took 20 years to master.

Outstanding Book!"—*Rusty Moore - Fitness Black Book - Seattle, WA*

A must for all martial artists

"As a dedicated martial artist for more than seven years, this book is exactly what I've been looking for.

For a while now I have trained with machines at my local gym to improve my muscle strength and power and get to the next level in my training. I always felt that the modern health club, technology based exercise jarred with my martial art though, which only required body movement.

Finally this book has come along. At last I can combine perfect body movement for martial skill with perfect body exercise for ultimate strength.

All fighting arts are based on body movement. This book is a complete textbook on how to max out your musclepower using only body movement, as different from dumbbells, machines or gadgets. For this reason it belongs on the bookshelf of every serious martial artist, male and female, young and old."—*Gino Cartier - Washington DC*

I've packed all of my other training books away!

"I read CC in one go. I couldn't put it down. I have purchased a lot of bodyweight training books in the past, and have always been pretty disappointed. They all seem to just have pictures of different exercises, and no plan whatsoever on how to implement them and progress with them. But not with this one. The information in this book is AWESOME! I like to have a clear, logical plan of progression to follow, and that is what this book gives. I have put all of my other training books away. CC is the only system I am going to follow. This is now my favorite training book ever!"—*Lyndan - Australia*

Brutal Elegance.

"I have been training and reading about training since I first joined the US Navy in the 1960s. I thought I'd seen everything the fitness world had to offer. Sometimes twice. But I was wrong. This book is utterly iconoclastic.

The author breaks down all conceivable body weight exercises into six basic movements, each designed to stimulate different vectors of the muscular system. These six are then elegantly and very intelligently broken into ten progressive techniques. You master one technique, and move on to the next.

The simplicity of this method belies a very powerful and complex training paradigm, reduced into an abstraction that obviously took many years of sweat and toil to develop.

Trust me. Nobody else worked this out. This approach is completely unique and fresh.

I have read virtually every calisthenics book printed in America over the last 40 years, and instruction like this can't be found anywhere, in any one of them. *Convict Conditioning* is head and shoulders above them all. In years to come, trainers and coaches will all be talking about 'progressions' and 'progressive calisthenics' and claim they've been doing it all along. But the truth is that Dragon Door bought it to you first. As with kettlebells, they were the trail blazers.

Who should purchase this volume? Everyone who craves fitness and strength should. Even if you don't plan to follow the routines, the book will make you think about your physical prowess, and will give even world class experts food for thought. At the very least if you find yourself on vacation or away on business without your barbells, this book will turn your hotel into a fully equipped gym.

I'd advise any athlete to obtain this work as soon as possible."—*Bill Oliver - Albany, NY, United States*

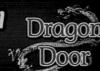

More Dragon Door Customer Acclaim for *Convict Conditioning*

Fascinating Reading and Real Strength

"Coach Wade's system is a real eye opener if you've been a lifetime iron junkie. Wanna find out how really strong (or weak) you are? Get this book and begin working through the 10 levels of the 6 power exercises...but some are downright humbling. If I were on a desert island with only one book on strength and conditioning this would be it. (Could I staple Pavel's "Naked Warrior" to the back and count them as one???!) Thanks Dragon Door for this innovative new author."—*Jon Schultheis, RKC (2005) - Keansburg, NJ*

Single best strength training book ever!

"I just turned 50 this year and I have tried a little bit of everything over the years: martial arts, swimming, soccer, cycling, free weights, weight machines, even yoga and Pilates. I started using *Convict Conditioning* right after it came out. I started from the beginning, like Coach Wade says, doing mostly step one or two for five out of the six exercises. I work out 3 to 5 times a week, usually for 30 to 45 minutes.

Long story short, my weight went up 14 pounds (I was not trying to gain weight) but my body fat percentage dropped two percent. That translates into approximately 19 pounds of lean muscle gained in two months! I've never gotten this kind of results with anything else I've ever done. Now I have pretty much stopped lifting weights for strength training. Instead, I lift once a week as a test to see how much stronger I'm getting without weight training. There are a lot of great strength training books in the world (most of them published by Dragon Door), but if I had to choose just one, this is the single best strength training book ever. BUY THIS BOOK. FOLLOW THE PLAN. GET AS STRONG AS YOU WANT. "—*Wayne - Decatur, GA*

Best bodyweight training book so far!

"I'm a martial artist and I've been training for years with a combination of weights and bodyweight training and had good results from both (but had the usual injuries from weight training). I prefer the bodyweight stuff though as it trains me to use my whole body as a unit, much more than weights do, and I notice the difference on the mat and in the ring. Since reading this book I have given the weights a break and focused purely on the bodyweight exercise progressions as described by 'Coach' Wade and my strength had increased more than ever before. So far I've built up to 12 strict one-leg squats each leg and 5 uneven pull ups each arm.

I've never achieved this kind of strength before - and this stuff builds solid muscle mass as well. It's very intense training. I am so confident in and happy with the results I'm getting that I've decided to train for a fitness/bodybuilding comp just using his techniques, no weights, just to show for real what kind of a physique these exercises can build. In sum, I cannot recommend 'Coach' Wade's book highly enough - it is by far the best of its kind ever!"—*Mark Robinson - Australia, currently living in South Korea*

A lifetime of lifting...and continued learning.

"I have been working out diligently since 1988 and played sports in high school and college before that. My stint in the Army saw me doing calisthenics, running, conditioning courses, forced marches, etc. There are many levels of strength and fitness. I have been as big as 240 in my powerlifting/strongman days and as low as 185-190 while in the Army. I think I have tried everything under the sun: the high intensity of Arthur Jones and Dr. Ken, the Super Slow of El Darden, and the brutality of Dinosaur Training Brooks Kubic made famous.

This is one of the BEST books I've ever read on real strength training which also covers other just as important aspects of health; like staying injury free, feeling healthy and becoming flexible. It's an excellent book. He tells you the why and the how with his progressive plan. This book is a GOLD MINE and worth 100 times what I paid for it!" —*Horst - Woburn, MA*

This book sets the standard, ladies and gentlemen

"It's difficult to describe just how much this book means to me. I've been training hard since I was in the RAF nearly ten years ago, and to say this book is a breakthrough is an understatement. How often do you really read something so new, so fresh? This book contains a complete new system of calisthenics drawn from American prison training methods. When I say 'system' I mean it. It's complete (rank beginner to expert), it's comprehensive (all the exercises and photos are here), it's graded (progressions from exercise to exercise are smooth and pre-determined) and it's totally original. Whether you love or hate the author, you have to listen to him. And you will learn something. This book just makes SENSE. In twenty years people will still be buying it."—*Andy McMann - Ponty, Wales, GB*

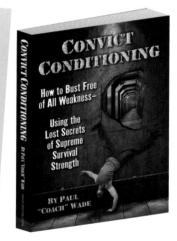

Convict Conditioning

How to Bust Free of All Weakness—Using the Lost Secrets of Supreme Survival Strength

By Paul "Coach" Wade

#B41 $39.95

eBook $19.95

Paperback 8.5 x 11 320 pages
191 photos, charts and illustrations

1 Beginner **2** Mid-Level **3** Advanced

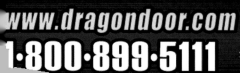

The Experts Give High Praise to
Convict Conditioning 2

"Coach Paul Wade has outdone himself. His first book *Convict Conditioning* is to my mind THE BEST book ever written on bodyweight conditioning. Hands down. Now, with the sequel *Convict Conditioning 2*, Coach Wade takes us even deeper into the subtle nuances of training with the ultimate resistance tool: our bodies.

In plain English, but with an amazing understanding of anatomy, physiology, kinesiology and, go figure, psychology, Coach Wade explains very simply how to work the smaller but just as important areas of the body such as the hands and forearms, neck and calves and obliques in serious functional ways.

His minimalist approach to exercise belies the complexity of his system and the deep insight into exactly how the body works and the best way to get from A to Z in the shortest time possible.

I got the best advice on how to strengthen the hard-to-reach extensors of the hand right away from this exercise Master I have ever seen. It's so simple but so completely functional I can't believe no one else has thought of it yet. Just glad he figured it out for me.

Paul teaches us how to strengthen our bodies with the simplest of movements while at the same time balancing our structures in the same way: simple exercises that work the whole body.

And just as simply as he did with his first book. His novel approach to stretching and mobility training is brilliant and fresh as well as his take on recovery and healing from injury. Sprinkled throughout the entire book are too-many-to-count insights and advice from a man who has come to his knowledge the hard way and knows exactly of what he speaks.

This book is, as was his first, an amazing journey into the history of physical culture disguised as a book on calisthenics. But the thing that Coach Wade does better than any before him is his unbelievable progressions on EVERY EXERCISE and stretch! He breaks things down and tells us EXACTLY how to proceed to get to whatever level of strength and development we want. AND gives us the exact metrics we need to know when to go to the next level.

Adding in completely practical and immediately useful insights into nutrition and the mindset necessary to deal not only with training but with life, makes this book a classic that will stand the test of time.

Bravo Coach Wade, Bravo." —Mark Reifkind, Master RKC, author of *Mastering the HardStyle Kettlebell Swing*

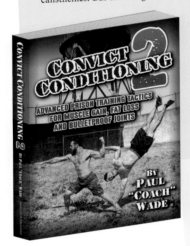

Convict Conditioning 2
Advanced Prison Training Tactics for Muscle Gain, Fat Loss and Bulletproof Joints
By Paul "Coach" Wade
#B59 $39.95
eBook $19.95
Paperback 8.5 x 11 354 pages
261 photos, charts and illustrations

Mid-Level

Advanced

"The overriding principle of *Convict Conditioning 2* is 'little equipment-big rewards'. For the athlete in the throwing and fighting arts, the section on Lateral Chain Training, Capturing the Flag, is a unique and perhaps singular approach to training the obliques and the whole family of side muscles. This section stood out to me as ground breaking and well worth the time and energy by anyone to review and attempt to complete. Literally, this is a new approach to lateral chain training that is well beyond sidebends and suitcase deadlifts.

The author's review of passive stretching reflects the experience of many of us in the field. But, his solution might be the reason I am going to recommend this work for everyone: The Trifecta. This section covers what the author calls The Functional Triad and gives a series of simple progressions to three holds that promise to oil your joints. It's yoga for the strength athlete and supports the material one would find, for example, in Pavel's *Loaded Stretching*.

I didn't expect to like this book, but I come away from it practically insisting that everyone read it. It is a strongman book mixed with yoga mixed with street smarts. I wanted to hate it, but I love it." —Dan John, author of *Don't Let Go* and co-author of *Easy Strength*

"I've been lifting weights for over 50 years and have trained in the martial arts since 1965. I've read voraciously on both subjects, and written dozens of magazine articles and many books on the subjects. This book and Wade's first, *Convict Conditioning*, are by far the most commonsense, information-packed, and result producing I've read. These books will truly change your life.

Paul Wade is a new and powerful voice in the strength and fitness arena, one that is commonsense, inspiring, and in your face. His approach to maximizing your body's potential is not the same old hackneyed material you find in every book and magazine piece that pictures steroid-bloated models screaming as they curl weights. Wade's stuff has been proven effective by hard men who don't tolerate fluff. It will work for you, too—guaranteed.

As an ex-cop, I've gone mano-y-mano with ex-cons that had clearly trained as Paul Wade suggests in his two *Convict Conditioning* books. While these guys didn't look like steroid-fueled bodybuilders (actually, there were a couple who did), all were incredibly lean, hard and powerful. Wade blows many commonly held beliefs about conditioning, strengthening, and eating out of the water and replaces them with result-producing information that won't cost you a dime." —Loren W. Christensen, author of *Fighting the Pain Resistant Attacker*, and many other titles

"*Convict Conditioning* is one of the most influential books I ever got my hands on. *Convict Conditioning 2* took my training and outlook on the power of bodyweight training to the 10th degree—from strengthening the smallest muscles in a maximal manner, all the way to using bodyweight training as a means of healing injuries that pile up from over 22 years of aggressive lifting.

I've used both *Convict Conditioning* and *Convict Conditioning 2* on myself and with my athletes. Without either of these books I can easily say that these boys would not be the BEASTS they are today. Without a doubt *Convict Conditioning 2* will blow you away and inspire and educate you to take bodyweight training to a whole NEW level." —Zach Even-Esh, Underground Strength Coach

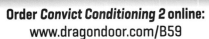

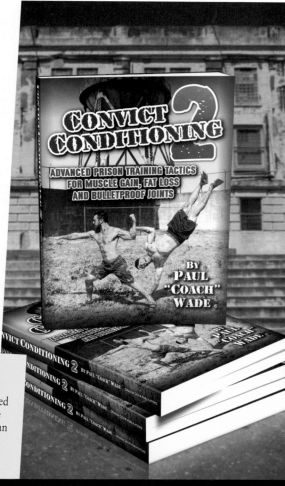

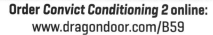

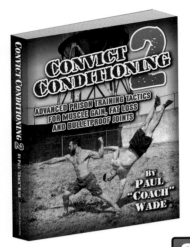

Convict Conditioning 2

Advanced Prison Training Tactics for Muscle Gain, Fat Loss and Bulletproof Joints

By Paul "Coach" Wade

#B59 $39.95

eBook $19.95

Paperback 8.5 x 11 354 pages
261 photos, charts and illustrations

2 Mid-Level

3 Advanced

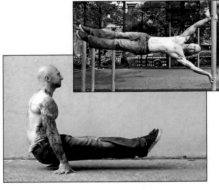

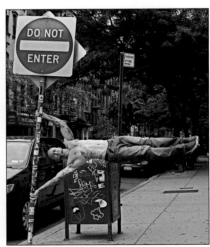

— TABLE OF CONTENTS —

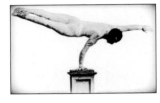

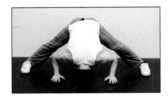
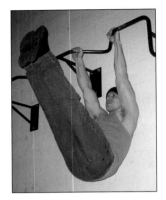
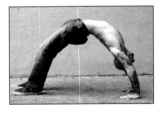
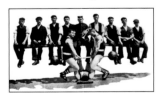
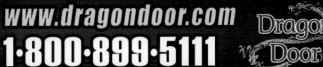

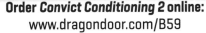

GET DYNAMIC, CHISELLED, POWER-JACK LEGS AND DEVELOP EXPLOSIVE LOWER-BODY STRENGTH—WITH PAUL "COACH" WADE'S ULTIMATE BODYWEIGHT SQUAT COURSE

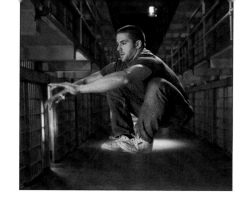

Paul Wade's *Convict Conditioning Ultimate Bodyweight Squat Course* explodes out of the cellblock to teach you in absolute detail how to progress from the ease of a simple shoulderstand squat—to the stunning "1-in-10,000" achievement of the prison-style one-leg squat. Ten progressive steps guide you to bodyweight squat mastery. Do it—and become a Bodyweight Squat Immortal.

This home-study course in ultimate survival strength comes replete with bonus material not available in **Paul Wade's** original *Convict Conditioning* book—and numerous key training tips that refine and expand on the original program.

A heavily and gorgeously-illustrated 80-plus-page manual gives you the entire film script to study at your leisure, with brilliant, precise photographs to remind you of the essential movements you absorbed in the DVD itself.

Paul Wade adds a bonus **Ten Commandments for Perfect Bodyweight Squats**—which is worth the price of admission alone. And there's the additional bonus of **5 major Variant** drills to add explosivity, fun and super-strength to your core practice.

Whatever you are looking for from your bodyweight squats—be it supreme functional strength, monstrous muscle growth or explosive leg power—it's yours for the progressive taking with *Convict Conditioning, Volume 2: The Ultimate Bodyweight Squat Course.*

WHY EVERY SELF-RESPECTING MAN WILL BE RELIGIOUS ABOUT HIS SQUATS...

Leg training is vital for every athlete. A well-trained, muscular upper body teetering around on skinny stick legs is a joke. Don't be that joke! The mighty squat is the answer to your prayers. Here's why:

- Squats train virtually every muscle in the lower body, from quads and glutes to hips, lower back and even hamstrings.

- Squat deep—as we'll teach you—and you will seriously increase your flexibility and ankle strength.

- All functional power is transmitted through the legs, so without strong, powerful legs you are *nothing*—that goes for running, jumping and combat sports as much as it does for lifting heavy stuff.

ARE YOU FAILING TO BUILD MONSTROUS LEGS FROM SQUATS—BECAUSE OF THESE MISTAKES?

Most trainees learn how to squat on two legs, and then make the exercise harder by slapping a barbell across their back. In prison, this way of adding strength wasn't always available, so cell trainees developed ways of progressing using only bodyweight versus gravity. The best way to do this is to learn how to squat all the way down to the ground and back up on just one leg.

Not everybody who explores prison training will have the dedication and drive to achieve strength feats like the one-arm pullup, but the legs are much stronger than the arms. If you put in the time and work hard, the one-leg squat will be within the reach of almost every athlete who pays their dues.

But the one-leg squat still requires very powerful muscles and tendons, so you don't want to jump into one-leg squatting right away. You need to build the joint strength and muscle to safely attempt this great exercise. Discover how to do that safely, using ten steps, ten progressively harder squat exercises.

IN THE STRENGTH GAME, FOOLS RUSH IN WHERE ANGELS FEAR TO TREAD

The wise old Chinese man shouted to his rickshaw driver: "Slow down, young man, I'm in a hurry!" If ever a warning needed to be shouted to our nation of compulsive strength-addicts, this would be it. You see them everywhere: the halt, the lame, the jacked-up, the torn, the pain-ridden—the former glory-seekers who have been reduced to sad husks of their former selves by rushing helter-skelter into heavy lifting without having first built a firm foundation.

Paul Wade reveals the ten key points of perfect squat form. The aspects of proper form apply to all your squats, and they'll not only unlock the muscle and power-building potential of each rep you do, but they'll also keep you as safe as you can be.

Bodyweight training is all about improving strength and health, not building up a list of injuries or aches and pains. They are so fundamental, we call them the Ten Commandments of good squat form.

Obey the Ten Commandments, follow the brilliantly laid out progressions religiously and you simply CANNOT fail to get stronger and stronger and stronger and stronger and stronger—surely, safely and for as long as you live…

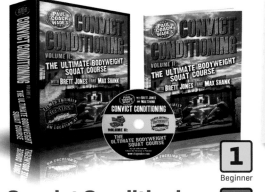
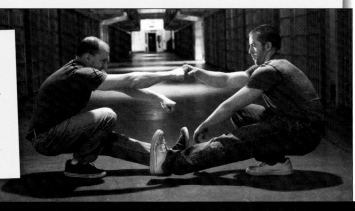
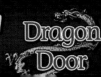

GET A ROCK-HARD, BRUTISHLY POWERFUL UPPER FRAME AND ACHIEVE ELITE-LEVEL STRENGTH— WITH PAUL "COACH" WADE'S PRISON-STYLE PUSHUP PROGRAM

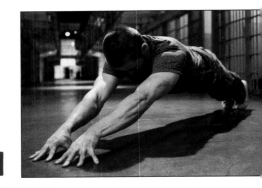

Paul Wade's *Convict Conditioning* system represents the ultimate distillation of hard-core prison bodyweight training's most powerful methods. What works was kept. What didn't, was slashed away. When your life is on the line, you're not going to mess with less than the absolute best. Many of these older, very potent solitary training systems have been on the verge of dying, as convicts begin to gain access to weights, and modern "bodybuilding thinking" floods into the

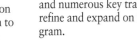

prisons. Thanks to Paul Wade, these ultimate strength survival secrets have been saved for posterity. And for you…

Filmed entirely—and so appropriately—on "The Rock", Wade's *Convict Conditioning Prison Pushup Series* explodes out of the cellblock to teach you in absolute detail how to progress from the ease of a simple wall pushup—to the stunning "1-in-10,000" achieve-

ment of the prison-style one-arm pushup. Ten progressive steps guide you to pushup mastery. Do it—and become a Pushup God.

This home-study course in ultimate survival strength comes replete with bonus material not available in **Paul Wade's** original *Convict Conditioning* book— and numerous key training tips that refine and expand on the original program.

A heavily and gorgeously-illustrated 80-plus-page manual gives you the entire film script to study at your leisure, with brilliant, precise photographs to remind you of the essential movements you absorbed in the DVD itself.

Paul Wade adds a bonus **Ten Commandments for Perfect Pushups**—which is worth the price of admission alone. And there's the additional bonus of **5 major Variant drills** to add explosivity, fun and super-strength to your core practice.

Whatever you are looking for from your pushups—be it supreme functional strength, monstrous muscle growth or explosive upper-body power—it's yours for the progressive taking with *Convict Conditioning, Volume 1: The Prison Pushup Series.*

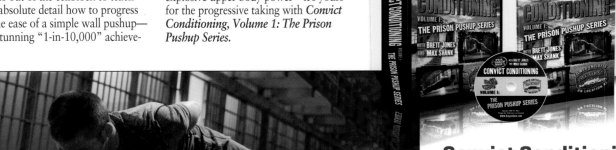

Convict Conditioning
Volume 1: The Prison Pushup Series
By Paul "Coach" Wade featuring Brett Jones and Max Shank
#DV083 $69.95
DVD 59 minutes with full color Companion Manual, 88 pages

1 Beginner
2 Mid-Level
3 Advanced

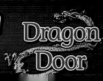

DEMONIC ABS ARE A MAN'S BEST FRIEND—DISCOVER HOW TO SEIZE A SIX-PACK FROM HELL AND OWN THE WORLD... LEG RAISES

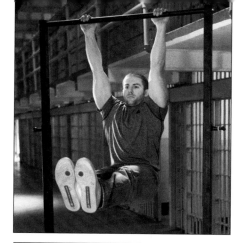

Paul Wade's *Convict Conditioning 3, Leg Raises: Six Pack from Hell* teaches you in absolute detail how to progress from the ease of a simple Knee Tuck—to the magnificent, "1-in-1,000" achievement of the Hanging Straight Leg Raise. Ten progressive steps guide you to inevitable mastery of this ultimate abs exercise. Do it, seize the knowledge—but beware—the Gods will be jealous!

This home-study course in ultimate survival strength comes replete with bonus material not available in **Paul Wade's** original *Convict Conditioning* book—and numerous key training tips that refine and expand on the original program.

Prowl through the heavily and gorgeously-illustrated 80-plus-page manual and devour the entire film script at your animal leisure. Digest the brilliant, precise photographs and reinforce the raw benefits you absorbed from the DVD.

Paul Wade adds a bonus **Ten Commandments for Perfect Bodyweight Squats**—which is worth the price of admission alone. And there's the additional bonus of **4 major Variant drills** to add explosivity, fun and super-strength to your core practice.

Whatever you are looking for when murdering your abs—be it a fist-breaking, rock-like shield of impenetrable muscle, an uglier-is-more-beautiful set of rippling abdominal ridges, or a monstrous injection of lifting power—it's yours for the progressive taking with *Convict Conditioning, Volume 3, Leg Raises: Six Pack from Hell*

PRISON-STYLE MID-SECTION TRAINING—FOR AN ALL SHOW AND ALL GO PHYSIQUE

When convicts train their waists, they want real,

noticeable results—and by "results" we don't mean that they want cute, tight little defined abs. We mean that they want thick, strong, muscular midsections. They want *functionally* powerful abs and hips they can use for heavy lifting, kicking, and brawling. They want guts so strong from their training that it actually hurts an attacker to punch them in the belly. Prison abs aren't about all show, no go—a prison-built physique has to be all show and all go. Those guys don't just want six-packs—they want six-packs from Hell.

And, for the first time, we're going to show you how these guys get what they want. We're not going to be using sissy machines or easy isolation exercises—we're going straight for the old school secret weapon for gut training; progressive leg raises.

If you want a six-pack from Hell, the first thing you need to do is focus your efforts. If a weightlifter wanted a very thick, powerful chest in a hurry, he wouldn't spread his efforts out over a dozen exercises and perform them gently all day long. No—he'd pick just one exercise, probably the bench press, and just focus on getting stronger and stronger on that lift until he was monstrously strong. When he reached this level, and his pecs were thick slabs of meat, only then would he maybe begin sculpting them with minor exercises and higher reps.

It's no different if you want a mind-blowing midsection. Just pick one exercise that hits all the muscles in the midsection—the hip flexors, the abs, the intercostals, the obliques—then blast it.

And the one exercise we're going to discover is the best midsection exercise known to man, and the most popular amongst soldiers, warriors, martial artists and prison athletes since men started working out—the leg raise.

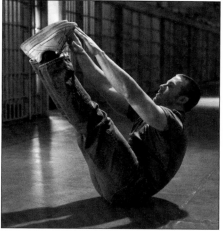

You'll discover ten different leg raise movements, each one a little harder than the last. You'll learn how to get the most out of each of these techniques, each of these ten steps, before moving up to the next step. By the time you get through all ten steps and you're working with the final Master Step of the leg raise series, you'll have a solid, athletic, stomach made of steel, as well as powerful hips and a ribcage armored with dense muscle. You'll have abs that would've made Bruce Lee take notice!

THE TEN COMMANDMENTS YOU MUST OBEY TO EARN A REAL MONSTER OF AN ATHLETIC CORE

Paul Wade gives you ten key points, the "Ten Commandments" of leg raises, that will take your prison-style core training from just "okay" to absolutely phenomenal. We want the results to be so effective that they'll literally shock you. This kind of accelerated progress can be achieved, but if you want to achieve it you better listen carefully to these ten key pointers you'll discover with the DVD.

Bodyweight mastery is a lot like high-level martial arts. It's more about *principles* than individual techniques. Really study and absorb these principles, and you'll be on your way to a six-pack from Hell in no time.

The hanging straight leg raise, performed strictly and for reps, is the Gold Standard of abdominal strength techniques. Once you're at the level where you can throw out sets of twenty to thirty rock solid reps of this exercise, your abs will be thick and strong, but more importantly, they'll be functional—not just a pretty six-pack, but a real monster of an athletic core, which is

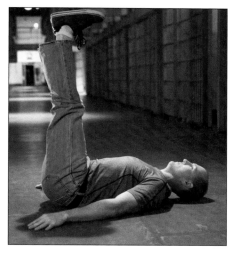

capable of developing high levels of force.

Hanging will work your serratus and intercostals, making these muscles stand out like fingers, and your obliques and flank muscles will be tight and strong from holding your hips in place. Your lumbar spine will achieve a gymnastic level of flexibility, like fluid steel, and your chances of back pain will be greatly reduced.

The bottom line: If you want to be stronger and more athletic than the next guy, you need the edge that straight leg raises can give you.

ERECT TWIN PYTHONS OF COILED BEEF UP YOUR SPINE AND DEVELOP EXTREME, EXPLOSIVE RESILIENCE—WITH THE DYNAMIC POWER AND FLEXIBLE STRENGTH OF ADVANCED BRIDGING

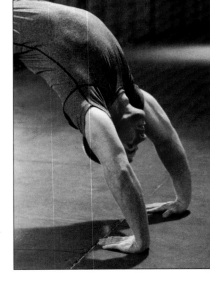

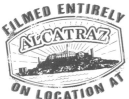

Paul Wade's *Convict Conditioning* system represents the ultimate distillation of hardcore prison bodyweight training's most powerful methods. What works was kept. What didn't, was slashed away. When your life is on the line, you're not going to mess with less than the absolute best. Many of these older, very potent solitary training systems have been on the verge of dying, as convicts begin to gain access to weights, and modern "bodybuilding thinking" floods into the prisons. Thanks to Paul Wade, these ultimate strength survival secrets have been saved for posterity. And for you…

Filmed entirely—and so appropriately— on "The Rock", Wade's *Convict Conditioning Volume 4, Advanced Bridging: Forging an Iron Spine* explodes out of the cellblock to teach you in absolute detail how to progress from the relative ease of a Short Bridge—to the stunning, "1-in-1,000" achievement of the Stand-to-Stand Bridge. Ten progressive steps guide you to inevitable mastery of this ultimate exercise for an unbreakable back.

This home-study course in ultimate survival strength comes replete with bonus material not available in **Paul Wade's** original *Convict Conditioning* book—and numerous key training tips that refine and expand on the original program.

Prowl through the heavily and gorgeously-illustrated 80-plus-page manual and devour the entire film script at your animal leisure. Digest the brilliant, precise photographs and reinforce the raw benefits you absorbed from the DVD.

Paul Wade adds a bonus **Ten Commandments for Perfect Bridges**— which is worth the price of admission alone. And there's the additional bonus of **4 major Variant drills** to add explosivity, fun and super-strength to your core practice.

Whatever you are looking for from your pushups—be it supreme functional strength, monstrous muscle growth or explosive upper-body power—it's yours for the progressive taking with *Convict Conditioning Volume 4: Advanced Bridging: Forging an Iron Spine.*

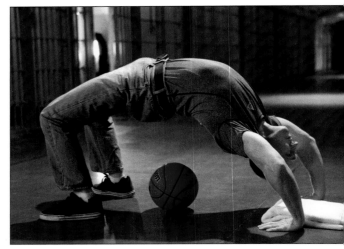

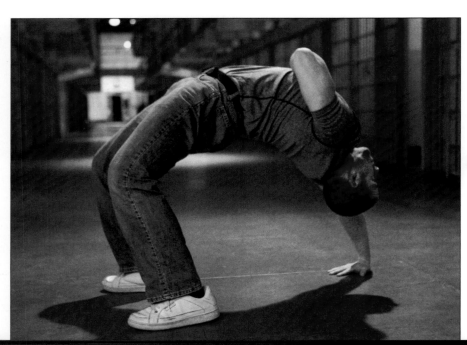

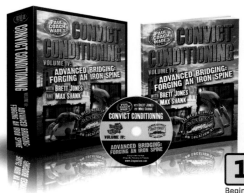

Convict Conditioning
Volume 4: Advanced Bridging: Forging an Iron Spine
By Paul "Coach" Wade featuring Brett Jones and Max Shank
#DV087 $59.95
DVD 59 minutes with full color Companion Manual, 88 pages

1 Beginner

2 Mid-Level

3 Advanced

TAP INTO THE DORMANT ANCESTRAL POWER OF THE MIGHTY PULLUP—
TO DEVELOP A MASSIVE UPPER BACK, STEEL-TENDON ARMS, ETCHED ABS AND AGILE SURVIVAL STRENGTH

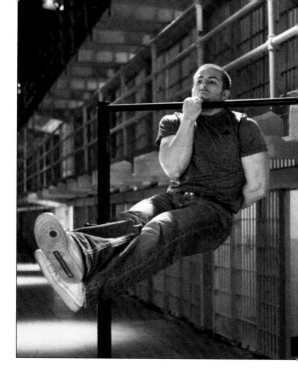

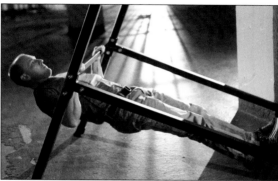

P aul Wade's *Convict Conditioning* system represents the ultimate distillation of hardcore prison bodyweight training's most powerful methods. What works was kept. What didn't, was slashed away. When your life is on the line, you're not going to mess with less than the absolute best. Many of these older, very potent solitary training systems have been on the verge of dying, as convicts begin to gain access to weights, and modern "bodybuilding thinking" floods into the prisons. Thanks to Paul Wade, these ultimate strength survival secrets have been saved for posterity. And for you...

Filmed entirely—and so appropriately— on "The Rock", Wade's *Convict Conditioning Volume 5, Maximum Strength: The One-Arm Pullup Series* explodes out of the cellblock to teach you in absolute detail how to progress from the relative ease of a Vertical Pull—to the stunning, "1-in-1,000" achievement of the One-Arm Pullup. Ten progressive steps guide you to inevitable mastery of this ultimate exercise for supreme upper body survival strength.

This home-study course in ultimate survival strength comes replete with bonus material not available in **Paul Wade's** original *Convict Conditioning* book—and numerous key training tips that refine and expand on the original program.

Prowl through the heavily and gorgeously-illustrated 80-plus-page manual and devour the entire film script at your animal leisure. Digest the brilliant, precise photographs and reinforce the raw benefits you absorbed from the DVD.

Paul Wade adds a bonus **Ten Commandments for Perfect Pullups**—which is worth the price of admission alone. And there's the additional bonus of **4 major Variant drills** to add explosivity, fun and super-strength to your core practice.

Whatever you are looking for from your pullups—be it agile survival strength, arms of steel, a massive upper back with flaring lats, Popeye Biceps or gape-inducing abs—it's yours for the progressive taking with *Convict Conditioning Volume 5, Maximum Strength: The One-Arm Pullup Series.*

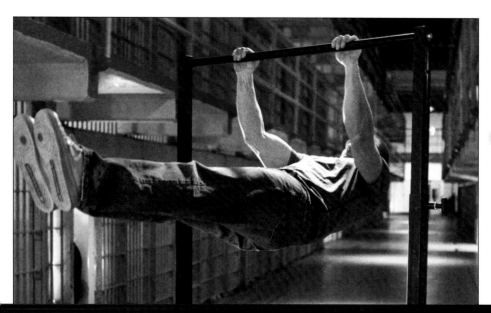

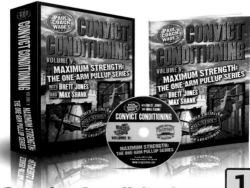

Convict Conditioning

Volume 5: Maximum Strength: The One-Arm Pullup Series
By Paul "Coach" Wade featuring Brett Jones and Max Shank
#DV088 $59.95
DVD 59 minutes with full color Companion Manual, 88 pages

1 Beginner

2 Mid-Level

3 Advanced

Al Kavadlo's Progressive Plan for Primal Body Power

How to Build Explosive Strength and a Magnificent Physique—Using Bodyweight Exercise Only

What is more satisfying than owning a primally powerful, functionally forceful and brute-strong body? A body that packs a punch. A body that commands attention with its etched physique, coiled muscle and proud confidence…A body that can PERFORM at the highest levels of physical accomplishment…

Well, both **Al Kavadlo**—the author of *Pushing the Limits!*—and his brother **Danny**, are supreme testaments to the primal power of body culture done the old-school, ancient way—bare-handed, with your body only. The brothers Kavadlo walk the bodyweight talk—and then some. The proof is evident on every page of *Pushing the Limits!*

Your body is your temple. Protect and strengthen your temple by modeling the methods of the exercise masters. Al Kavadlo has modeled the masters and has the "temple" to show for it. Follow Al's progressive plan for primal body power within the pages of *Pushing the Limits!*—follow in the footsteps of the great bodyweight exercise masters— and you too can build the explosive strength and possess the magnificent physique you deserve.

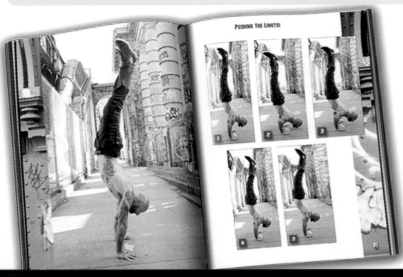

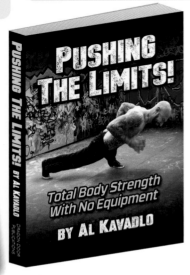

Pushing the Limits!
Total Body Strength With No Equipment
By Al Kavadlo
#B69 $39.95
eBook $19.95
Paperback 8.5 x 11   224 pages
240 photos

1 Beginner   **2** Mid-Level   **3** Advanced

Stretching and Flexibility Secrets To Help Unlock Your Body—Be More Mobile, More Athletic, More Resilient And Far Stronger...

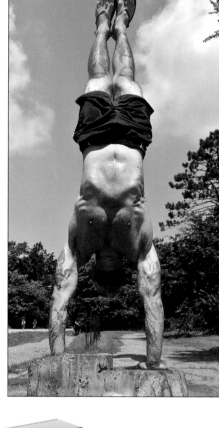

"The ultimate bodyweight mobility manual is here! Al Kavadlo's previous two Dragon Door books, *Raising the Bar* and *Pushing the Limits*, are the most valuable bodyweight strength training manuals in the world. But strength without mobility is meaningless. Al has used his many years of training and coaching to fuse bodyweight disciplines such as yoga, martial arts, rehabilitative therapy and bar athletics into the ultimate calisthenics stretching compendium. *Stretching your Boundaries* belongs on the shelf of any serious athlete—it's bodyweight mobility dynamite!"
—"COACH" PAUL WADE, author of *Convict Conditioning*

"In this book, Al invites you to take a deeper look at the often overlooked, and sometimes demonized, ancient practice of static stretching. He wrestles with many of the questions, dogmas and flat out lies about stretching that have plagued the fitness practitioner for at least the last decade. And finally he gives you a practical guide to static stretching that will improve your movement, performance, breathing and life. In *Stretching Your Boundaries,* you'll sense Al's deep understanding and love for the human body. Thank you Al, for helping to bring awareness to perhaps the most important aspect of physical education and fitness."
—ELLIOTT HULSE, creator of the **Grow Stronger** method

"An absolutely masterful follow up to *Raising The Bar* and *Pushing The Limits, Stretching Your Boundaries* really completes the picture. Both easy to understand and fully applicable, Al's integration of traditional flexibility techniques with his own unique spin makes this a must have. The explanation of how each stretch will benefit your calisthenics practice is brilliant. Not only stunning in its color and design, this book also gives you the true feeling of New York City, both gritty and euphoric, much like Al's personality."
—MIKE FITCH, creator of **Global Bodyweight Training**

"Stretching Your Boundaries is a terrific resource that will unlock your joints so you can build more muscle, strength and athleticism. Al's passion for human performance radiates in this beautifully constructed book. Whether you're stiff as a board, or an elite gymnast, this book outlines the progressions to take your body and performance to a new level."
—CHAD WATERBURY, M.S., author of *Huge in a Hurry*

"Al Kavadlo has done it again! He's created yet another incredible resource that I wish I had twenty years ago. Finding great material on flexibility training that actually enhances your strength is like trying to find a needle in a haystack. But look no further, because *Stretching Your Boundaries* is exactly what you need."
—JASON FERRUGGIA, Strength Coach

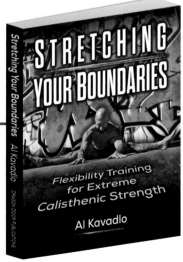

Stretching Your Boundaries
Flexibility Training for Extreme Calisthenic Strength
By Al Kavadlo
#B73 $39.95
eBook $19.95
Paperback 8.5 x 11   214 pages
235 photos

Beginner   Mid-Level   Advanced

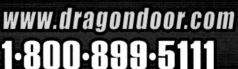

Go Beyond Mere "Toughness"— When You Master The Art of Bar Athletics and Sculpt the Ultimate in Upper Body Physiques

> "*Raising the Bar* is very likely the most important book on strength and conditioning to be published in the last fifty years. If you only ever get your hands on one training manual in your life, make it this one. Buy it, read it, use it. This book has the power to transform you into the ultimate bar athlete." —**Paul "Coach" Wade**, author of *Convict Conditioning*

Raising the Bar
The Definitive Guide to Bar Calisthenics
By Al Kavadlo
#B63 $39.95   eBook $19.95
224 pages, 330 Photos

1 Beginner **2** Mid-Level **3** Advanced

Raising the Bar breaks down every type of exercise you can do with a pull-up bar. From the basic two arm hang, to the mighty muscle-up, all the way to the elusive one arm pull-up, "bar master" Al Kavadlo takes you step by expert step through everything you need to do to build the chiseled frame you've always wanted.

Whether you're a die-hard calisthenics enthusiast or just looking to get in the best shape of your life, *Raising the Bar* will meet all your expectations—and then some!

The message is clear: you can earn yourself a stunning upper body with just 3 basic moves and 1 super-simple, yet amazingly versatile tool.

And what's even better, this 3 + 1 formula for upper body magnificence hides enough variety to keep you challenged and surging to new heights for a lifetime of cool moves and ever-tougher progressions!

Cast in the "concrete jungle" of urban scaffolding and graffiti-laden, blasted walls—and sourced from iconic bar-athlete destinations like Tompkins Square Park, NYC—*Raising the Bar* rears up to grab you by the throat and hurl you into an inspiring new vision of what the human body can achieve. Embrace Al Kavadlo's vision, pick up the challenge, share the Quest, follow directions—and the Holy Grail of supreme upper body fitness is yours for the taking.

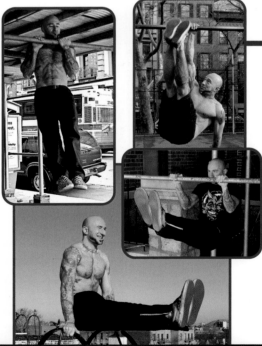

"With *Raising the Bar*, Al Kavadlo has put forth the perfect primal pull-up program. Al's progressions and demonstrations make even the most challenging exercises attainable. Anyone who is serious about pull-ups should read this book."—**Mark Sisson**, author of *The Primal Blueprint*.

A Kick Ass Encyclopedia of Bodyweight Exercises

"Al Kavadlo has put together a kick ass encyclopedia of the most powerful and most commonly used bodyweight exercises amongst the various groups of bodyweight masters.

From the most simple form of each exercise progressing to the most challenging form of each exercise, Al covers it. As a Coach and bodyweight training addict I loved all the variations shown. This book is far beyond just pull ups and there are countless exercises for upper body and abs. Al covers what is probably EVERY exercise he knows of, uses and teaches others, breaking down proper techniques, regressions and progressions. This is HUGE for the trainers out there who do NOT know how to adapt bodyweight exercises to each individual's fitness level.

If you're a fan of bodyweight training, between this book and *Convict Conditioning* you can turn your body into a deadly weapon!!!" —**Zach Even-Esh**, Manasquan, NJ

"Al has put together the companion manual for all the crazy bar calisthenics videos that you find yourself watching over and over again—a much needed resource. Within this book is a huge volume of bar exercises that will keep your pullup workouts fresh for years, and give you some insane goals to shoot for."
—**Max Shank**, Senior RKC

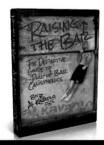

Raising the Bar
The Definitive Guide to Bar Calisthenics
DVD with Al Kavadlo
#DV090 $29.95
224 pages, 330 Photos

C-MASS

How To Maximize Muscle Growth Using Bodyweight-Only Training

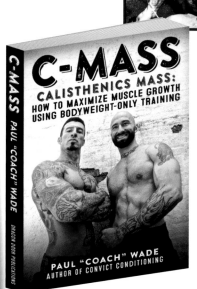

Is it really possible to add significant extra muscle-bulk to your frame using bodyweight exercise only? The answer, according to calisthenics guru and bestselling *Convict Conditioning* author *Paul Wade*, is a resounding Yes. Legendary strongmen and savvy modern bodyweight bodybuilders both, have added stacks of righteous beef to their physiques—using just the secrets *Paul Wade* reveals in this bible-like guide to getting as strong AND as big as you could possibly want, using nothing but your own body.

Paul Wade's trenchant, visceral style blazes with hard-won body culture insight, tactics, strategies and tips for the ultimate blueprint for getting huge naturally without free weights, machine supplements or—God forbid—steroids. With *C-Mass*, *Paul Wade* further cements his position as the preeminent modern authority on how to build extraordinary power and strength with bodyweight exercise only.

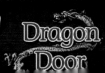

C-MASS
Calisthenics Mass: How To Maximize Muscle Growth Using Bodyweight-Only Training
By Paul "Coach" Wade
#B75 $24.95
eBook $9.95
Paperback 8.5 x 11 135 pages
135 photos

 1 Beginner   **2** Mid-Level   **3** Advanced

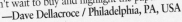

Get Harder, Stronger, More Powerful and Ripped to Shreds—with PCC, the World's Premier Bodyweight Exercise Training Program

Based on the teachings of Convict Conditioning founder, PAUL WADE… led by AL and DANNY KAVADLO

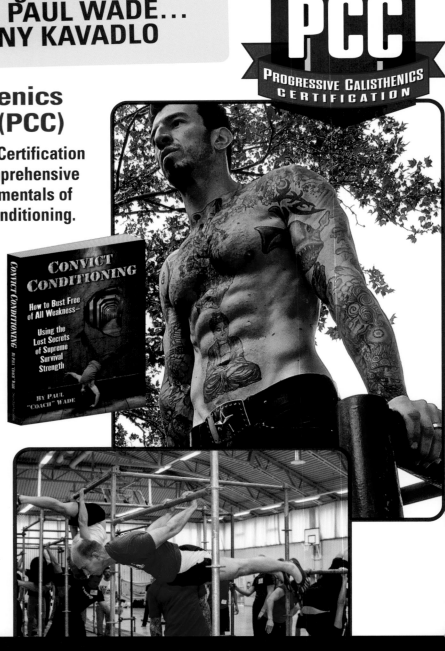

The Progressive Calisthenics Certification Workshop (PCC)

Dragon Door's Progressive Calisthenics Certification (PCC) provides you the world's most comprehensive training in the core principles and fundamentals of bodyweight exercise for strength and conditioning.

Master the cutting-edge bodyweight exercise progressions developed by **Convict Conditioning** founder **Paul Wade**—and earn the right to teach this acclaimed system to athletes, martial artists, trainers, coaches and all men and women dedicated to the cultivation of supreme strength and rugged toughness.

→ **Discover how** to generate tigrish power, enhance your coordination and balance, protect your joints, transform your physique, build steel-like tendon integrity and blowtorch fat from your body.

→ **Boost your value** as a coach or personal trainer. Not only are the movements extraordinarily cool— and adjustable to any skill level—they are also amongst the most effective, functional techniques on earth.

→ **The PCC** represents the *ultimate bodyweight cert,* and whatever your field or specialization—from strength training to rehab, bodybuilding to team sports—you will come away from this three-day cert with vast resources of training knowledge unavailable anywhere else.

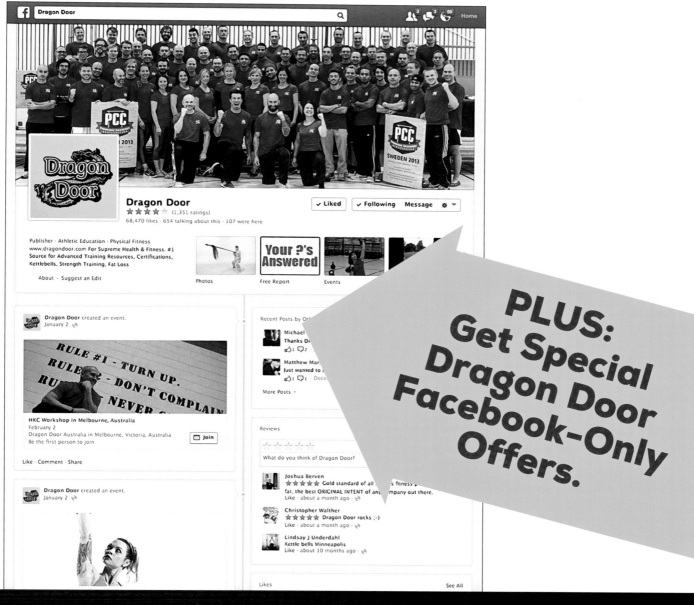

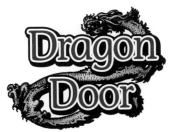

1·800·899·5111
24 HOURS A DAY • FAX YOUR ORDER (866) 280-7619
ORDERING INFORMATION

Telephone Orders For faster service you may place your orders by calling Toll Free 24 hours a day, 7 days a week, 365 days per year. When you call, please have your credit card ready.

Customer Service Questions? Please call us between 9:00am– 11:00pm EST

Monday to Friday at 1-800-899-5111. Local and foreign customers call 513-346-4160 for orders and customer service

100% One-Year Risk-Free Guarantee. If you are not completely satisfied with any product—we'll be happy to give you a prompt exchange,

credit, or refund, as you wish. Simply return your purchase to us, and please let us know why you were dissatisfied—it will help us to provide better products and services in the future. *Shipping and handling fees are non-refundable.*

VISA · MasterCard · AMERICAN EXPRESS Cards · DISCOVER NOVUS

Complete and mail with full payment to: Dragon Door Publications, 5 County Road B East, Suite 3, Little Canada, MN 55117

Please print clearly
Sold To: A

Name_____

Street _____

City _____

State _____ Zip _____

Day phone*_____
* Important for clarifying questions on orders

Please print clearly
SHIP TO: *(Street address for delivery)*   B

Name_____

Street _____

City _____

State _____ Zip _____

Email _____

Warning to foreign customers:
The Customs in your country may or may not tax or otherwise charge you an additional fee for goods you receive. Dragon Door Publications is charging you only for U.S. handling and international shipping. Dragon Door Publications is in no way responsible for any additional fees levied by Customs, the carrier or any other entity.

ITEM #	QTY.	ITEM DESCRIPTION	ITEM PRICE	A OR B	TOTAL

HANDLING AND SHIPPING CHARGES • NO COD'S
Total Amount of Order Add (Excludes kettlebells and kettlebell kits):

$00.00 to 29.99	**Add $6.00**	$100.00 to 129.99	**Add $14.00**
$30.00 to 49.99	**Add $7.00**	$130.00 to 169.99	**Add $16.00**
$50.00 to 69.99	**Add $8.00**	$170.00 to 199.99	**Add $18.00**
$70.00 to 99.99	**Add $11.00**	$200.00 to 299.99	**Add $20.00**
		$300.00 and up	**Add $24.00**

Canada and Mexico add $6.00 to US charges. All other countries, flat rate, double US Charges. See Kettlebell section for Kettlebell Shipping and handling charges.

Total of Goods	
Shipping Charges	
Rush Charges	
Kettlebell Shipping Charges	
OH residents add 6.5% sales tax	
MN residents add 6.5% sales tax	
TOTAL ENCLOSED	

METHOD OF PAYMENT ☐ CHECK ☐ M.O. ☐ MASTERCARD ☐ VISA ☐ DISCOVER ☐ AMEX

Account No. *(Please indicate all the numbers on your credit card)*   EXPIRATION DATE

☐☐☐☐ ☐☐☐☐ ☐☐☐☐ ☐☐☐☐   ☐☐/☐☐

Day Phone: (____)_____

Signature: _____   **Date:** _____

NOTE: *We ship best method available for your delivery address. Foreign orders are sent by air. Credit card or International M.O. only. For* **RUSH** *processing of your order, add an additional $10.00 per address. Available on money order & charge card orders only.*

Errors and omissions excepted. Prices subject to change without notice.

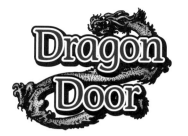

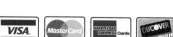

1·800·899·5111
24 HOURS A DAY • FAX YOUR ORDER (866) 280-7619
ORDERING INFORMATION

Telephone Orders For faster service you may place your orders by calling Toll Free 24 hours a day, 7 days a week, 365 days per year. When you call, please have your credit card ready.

Customer Service Questions? Please call us between 9:00am– 11:00pm EST

Monday to Friday at 1-800-899-5111. Local and foreign customers call 513-346-4160 for orders and customer service

100% One-Year Risk-Free Guarantee. If you are not completely satisfied with any product—we'll be happy to give you a prompt exchange,

credit, or refund, as you wish. Simply return your purchase to us, and please let us know why you were dissatisfied—it will help us to provide better products and services in the future. *Shipping and handling fees are non-refundable.*

Complete and mail with full payment to: Dragon Door Publications, 5 County Road B East, Suite 3, Little Canada, MN 55117

Please print clearly
Sold To: A

Name_____

Street _____

City _____

State _____ Zip _____

Day phone*_____
* Important for clarifying questions on orders

Please print clearly
SHIP TO: *(Street address for delivery)*   B

Name_____

Street _____

City _____

State _____ Zip _____

Email _____

Warning to foreign customers:
The Customs in your country may or may not tax or otherwise charge you an additional fee for goods you receive. Dragon Door Publications is charging you only for U.S. handling and international shipping. Dragon Door Publications is in no way responsible for any additional fees levied by Customs, the carrier or any other entity.

Item #	Qty.	Item Description	Item Price	A or B	Total

HANDLING AND SHIPPING CHARGES • NO COD'S
Total Amount of Order Add (Excludes kettlebells and kettlebell kits):

$00.00 to 29.99	Add $6.00	$100.00 to 129.99	Add $14.00
$30.00 to 49.99	Add $7.00	$130.00 to 169.99	Add $16.00
$50.00 to 69.99	Add $8.00	$170.00 to 199.99	Add $18.00
$70.00 to 99.99	Add $11.00	$200.00 to 299.99	Add $20.00
		$300.00 and up	Add $24.00

Canada and Mexico add $6.00 to US charges. All other countries, flat rate, double US Charges. See Kettlebell section for Kettlebell Shipping and handling charges.

Total of Goods	
Shipping Charges	
Rush Charges	
Kettlebell Shipping Charges	
OH residents add 6.5% sales tax	
MN residents add 6.5% sales tax	
Total Enclosed	

METHOD OF PAYMENT ❑ Check ❑ M.O. ❑ Mastercard ❑ Visa ❑ Discover ❑ Amex

Account No. *(Please indicate all the numbers on your credit card)*   EXPIRATION DATE

☐☐☐☐ ☐☐☐☐ ☐☐☐☐ ☐☐☐☐   ☐☐/☐☐

Day Phone: (___) _____

Signature: _____ **Date:** _____

NOTE: *We ship best method available for your delivery address. Foreign orders are sent by air. Credit card or international M.O. only. For **RUSH** processing of your order, add an additional $10.00 per address. Available on money order & charge card orders only.*

Errors and omissions excepted. Prices subject to change without notice.

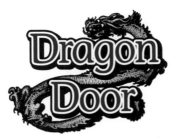

1·800·899·5111

24 HOURS A DAY • FAX YOUR ORDER (866) 280-7619

O R D E R I N G   I N F O R M A T I O N

Telephone Orders For faster service you may place your orders by calling Toll Free 24 hours a day, 7 days a week, 365 days per year. When you call, please have your credit card ready.

Customer Service Questions? Please call us between 9:00am– 11:00pm EST

Monday to Friday at 1-800-899-5111. Local and foreign customers call 513-346-4160 for orders and customer service

100% One-Year Risk-Free Guarantee. If you are not completely satisfied with any product—we'll be happy to give you a prompt exchange,

credit, or refund, as you wish. Simply return your purchase to us, and please let us know why you were dissatisfied— it will help us to provide better products and services in the future. *Shipping and handling fees are non-refundable.*

Complete and mail with full payment to: Dragon Door Publications, 5 County Road B East, Suite 3, Little Canada, MN 55117

Please print clearly

Sold To: **A**

Name_____

Street_____

City_____

State _____ Zip _____

Day phone*_____
* Important for clarifying questions on orders

Please print clearly

SHIP TO: *(Street address for delivery)*   **B**

Name_____

Street_____

City_____

State _____ Zip _____

Email_____

Warning to foreign customers:
The Customs in your country may or may not tax or otherwise charge you an additional fee for goods you receive. Dragon Door Publications is charging you only for U.S. handling and international shipping. Dragon Door Publications is in no way responsible for any additional fees levied by Customs, the carrier or any other entity.

Item #	Qty.	Item Description	Item Price	A or B	Total

HANDLING AND SHIPPING CHARGES • NO COD'S

Total Amount of Order Add (Excludes kettlebells and kettlebell kits):

$00.00 to 29.99	**Add $6.00**	**$100.00 to 129.99**	**Add $14.00**
$30.00 to 49.99	**Add $7.00**	**$130.00 to 169.99**	**Add $16.00**
$50.00 to 69.99	**Add $8.00**	**$170.00 to 199.99**	**Add $18.00**
$70.00 to 99.99	**Add $11.00**	**$200.00 to 299.99**	**Add $20.00**
		$300.00 and up	**Add $24.00**

Canada and Mexico add $6.00 to US charges. All other countries, flat rate, double US Charges. See Kettlebell section for Kettlebell Shipping and handling charges.

Total of Goods	
Shipping Charges	
Rush Charges	
Kettlebell Shipping Charges	
OH residents add 6.5% sales tax	
MN residents add 6.5% sales tax	
Total Enclosed	

METHOD OF PAYMENT ❑ Check ❑ M.O. ❑ Mastercard ❑ Visa ❑ Discover ❑ Amex

Account No. *(Please indicate all the numbers on your credit card)*   EXPIRATION DATE

☐☐☐☐ ☐☐☐☐ ☐☐☐☐ ☐☐☐☐   ☐☐/☐☐

Day Phone: (___)_____

Signature: _____ **Date:** _____

NOTE: *We ship best method available for your delivery address. Foreign orders are sent by air. Credit card or International M.O. only. For **RUSH** processing of your order, add an additional $10.00 per address. Available on money order & charge card orders only.*

Errors and omissions excepted. Prices subject to change without notice.

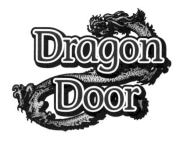

1·800·899·5111

24 HOURS A DAY • FAX YOUR ORDER (866) 280-7619

O R D E R I N G   I N F O R M A T I O N

Telephone Orders For faster service you may place your orders by calling Toll Free 24 hours a day, 7 days a week, 365 days per year. When you call, please have your credit card ready.

Customer Service Questions? Please call us between 9:00am– 11:00pm EST

Monday to Friday at 1-800-899-5111. Local and foreign customers call 513-346-4160 for orders and customer service

100% One-Year Risk-Free Guarantee. If you are not completely satisfied with any product—we'll be happy to give you a prompt exchange,

credit, or refund, as you wish. Simply return your purchase to us, and please let us know why you were dissatisfied— it will help us to provide better products and services in the future. *Shipping and handling fees are non-refundable.*

Complete and mail with full payment to: Dragon Door Publications, 5 County Road B East, Suite 3, Little Canada, MN 55117

Please print clearly

Sold To: A

Name_____

Street _____

City _____

State _____ Zip _____

Day phone*_____
* Important for clarifying questions on orders

Please print clearly

SHIP TO: *(Street address for delivery)*   B

Name_____

Street _____

City _____

State _____ Zip _____

Email _____

Warning to foreign customers:
The Customs in your country may or may not tax or otherwise charge you an additional fee for goods you receive. Dragon Door Publications is charging you only for U.S. handling and international shipping. Dragon Door Publications is in no way responsible for any additional fees levied by Customs, the carrier or any other entity.

ITEM #	QTY.	ITEM DESCRIPTION	ITEM PRICE	A OR B	TOTAL

HANDLING AND SHIPPING CHARGES • NO COD'S
Total Amount of Order Add (Excludes kettlebells and kettlebell kits):

$00.00 to 29.99	Add $6.00	$100.00 to 129.99	Add $14.00
$30.00 to 49.99	Add $7.00	$130.00 to 169.99	Add $16.00
$50.00 to 69.99	Add $8.00	$170.00 to 199.99	Add $18.00
$70.00 to 99.99	Add $11.00	$200.00 to 299.99	Add $20.00
		$300.00 and up	Add $24.00

Canada and Mexico add $6.00 to US charges. All other countries, flat rate, double US Charges. See Kettlebell section for Kettlebell Shipping and handling charges.

Total of Goods	
Shipping Charges	
Rush Charges	
Kettlebell Shipping Charges	
OH residents add 6.5% sales tax	
MN residents add 6.5% sales tax	
TOTAL ENCLOSED	

METHOD OF PAYMENT ❑ CHECK ❑ M.O. ❑ MASTERCARD ❑ VISA ❑ DISCOVER ❑ AMEX

Account No. *(Please indicate all the numbers on your credit card)*   EXPIRATION DATE

☐☐☐☐ ☐☐☐☐ ☐☐☐☐ ☐☐☐☐   ☐☐/☐☐

Day Phone: (___)_____

Signature: _____   **Date:** _____

NOTE: *We ship best method available for your delivery address. Foreign orders are sent by air. Credit card or international M.O. only. For* **RUSH** *processing of your order, add an additional $10.00 per address. Available on money order & charge card orders only.*

Errors and omissions excepted. Prices subject to change without notice.